THEY'RE NOT
JUST
DOGS AND CATS

Donald J. Calaceto, DVM
May 28, 2014

First published by Dog Ear Publishing
4010 W. 86th Street, Ste H
Indianapolis, IN 46268
www.dogearpublishing.net

dog ear
PUBLISHING

ISBN: 978-1-4575-1447-0

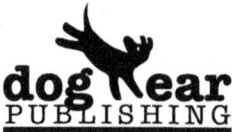

PREFACE

Writing this short book provided a sound method to trace the journey I have made in my professional and personal life. The following pages include select cases as they occurred in the last three years so that I had vivid memories to share. Time did not have the chance to alter my recollection of the facts. These cases discussed are exemplary of other cases I experienced over the past three decades briefly as an Equine and then mostly as a Small Animal Practitioner.

My personal life was only discussed to familiarize the reader somewhat with my persona, so that he or she could understand my intentions as a Veterinarian.

More than thirty years ago, I had great hopes that I would provide better services as a doctor than I had received as a dog owner in the late 1970's, when practitioners hesitated to treat my dog who was in urgent need of high quality veterinary care.

I have learned that the prevailing shortcomings in the delivery of high quality veterinary care are not due to the lack of genuine interest by the doctor. Instead, deficient veterinary care is due to an absence of government financial assistance and direction.

There is nothing I can do as a private practitioner except charity work to improve this situation that has been left unattended by the government. It's not enough to just care.

Just caring about your family, doesn't pay for their surgery or medicine either.

After thirty years in the veterinary community I find it very frustrating to continue practicing because of the lack of commitment to quality animal health care by the government and the constituent pet owners they represent. The national and state veterinary organizations have not expressed that we are in dire need of government intervention including financial assistance to guarantee quality veterinary health care.

I became a Veterinarian in hopes of making a difference. So far I have not made any difference, because the battlefront to improve veterinary health care is not at the hospital as I once thought.

Instead, the battlefront is with constituents and legislatures to convince them that laws must be enacted to improve pet owner, veterinary and government conduct. But before these laws can work, tax revenue needs to be appropriated and tax deductions allowed for pet owners to make veterinary care more affordable and accessible, and institutions, social services put in place by federal and state government to assist in the delivery, and payment of veterinary health care to stop animal suffering and cruelty.

This Book is dedicated to my present family including:
My mother, Giovanna Lamanuzzi Calaceto,
My daughters, Jillian, Abigail, Sara and Caroline
Their mother Mary Ellen Rago,
My sister Claudia Lynne Calaceto, and
My wife, LuAnn Skelly Calaceto
Whom have supported me in my effort
to raise awareness and begin a movement to remedy
The Veterinary Health Care Crisis

PART ONE

THE CRISIS

"I love the dog like she's one of the children, but 500.00 is a lot of money to spend. My husband has been out of work for 15 months. What should I do? The children come first." Why so much drama? Would you believe to try to make a convincing excuse not to spend money to nurse the dog back to health?

I said we accept any type of credit card so you can finance the work. "But is she suffering.?" I said I don't know I haven't examined her. How much will that cost? Forty eight dollars to examine her an come up with a plan for her care. Do the owners really care enough about preserving their pet's life? Maybe.

Webster defines care as to feel interest, concern or solicitude. Solicitude might be the most accurate word to describe how these people feel. Solicitude defined by Webster as an uneasiness of mind due to fear of future developments. In this case, if the dog receives the veterinary care required, the fear of imminent financial setback and the subsequent risk of loosing their home security is their greatest worry. In fact, our family pet's ailing health concerns even take a back seat to the repair work needed on our car. Should we spend money to help our family dog who is having trouble catching her breath, and who has not eaten and drank sufficiently in days to sustain life? What do you think?

Clearly, something needs to be done immediately. But if we wait long enough some of these animals will suffer and perish without treatment that may have been helpful if a diagnosis was attained after an examination and adequate diagnostics tools. What is the real reason why she didn't want to spend some money to try to keep the dog alive and well? This is a very disturbing question. One which I will try to answer in this book. Why try and fix it? It's cheaper to get a new one especially when you can get cheap shots and cheap spays and neuters by Low Cost Providers (LCP). Ultimately when the animal is finally seen weeks later DOA the owner will ask "Did she suffer?" Should I say yes, from neglect? To avoid this neglect, does that imply that I should offer free services or even free euthanasia for every potentially treatable animal that comes into the office, when the owner doesn't have or pretends not to have sufficient funds to properly diagnose their pets condition. Don't I have to live with my conscience after every one of these cases?

The fact is that in many cases, because they do not have sufficient funds, it is a struggle to convince many of them to spend enough to diagnose and treat their pet in hopes of attaining favorable results. Instead they often prefer to come up with the 190.00 as in this case to charge to their credit card for individual cremation.

Instead of spending an uncertain amount of money on their credit card to even diagnose their pets condition., they're more willing to spend less money to euthanize the animal and get the ashes back, and buy a replacement pet. I did not become a Veterinarian to assist these people with unwarranted euthanasia. I became a Veterinarian to strive to successfully diagnose and treat animals. Euthanasia should be a joint decision made between the doctor and patient based on the medical facts and a grave prognosis.

I never imagined that the practice of Veterinary Medicine to treat diseases was not a workable solution for many people. Why do many owners act as if the only time you bring pets to Veterinarians other than vaccinations and altering is to end their life ? Because the veterinary profession has allowed this perception to exist, because of pet owners financial limitations to pay for medical and surgical solutions. We are mostly able to help the medical and surgical cases that don't require extended hospitalization (beyond 3 days) i.e. non complicated gastrointestinal digestive and genitourinary diseases, dentals, simple orthopedic procedures, uncomplicated external tumor removals, and simple eye and ear surgery when charges usually do not exceed 750.00. Furthermore, let me emphasize simple. Anything that involves very careful and/or extensive home nursing care is not a acceptable plan either.

If given a second chance at youth, would I choose again to be a Veterinarian? I am afraid not.

This is how it all started.

Let's push the clock back to the mid 1970's. Back then I had a wonderful dog who I considered a large part of my life. We went just about everywhere together. Camping trips, long hikes as well as routine errands. At the age of seven she got terribly ill. She presented with bloody stools, inappetance, nausea and considerable lethargy. As it turned out, she would require extended hospitalization, but not for a definitive diagnosis or successful treatment. . All the veterinarians accept a Pakistani practitioner did not show an interest in taking her on as a patient.. Payment concerns did not even come up. He kept the dog at his office for a couple of weeks until she died. All he did was provide hospice care to my dog without ever rendering a diagnosis. Diagnostic tests were not performed to find a cause of her disease. Maybe if an effort was made to find a specific cause and intensive care provided she may have survived.

At least in human medicine you get a cause of disease when you hear about a person dying receiving hospice care.

Those people close to me knew how disappointed I was with the loss of my companion and what I thought was the lack of expertise and/or sincere interest by veterinarians. My father and I went up into the attic to uncover a solid wood door and proceeded to design and construct a casket. Yes, I said a casket.

It was our way of showing respect for her. I Then dug a hole on our bird path below frost line to bury my friend who wasn't given the opportunity she deserved to be diagnosed and treated by all the veterinarians that I asked for assistance.

After this experience, I began to consider this profession as my life's work, because I hoped that the answer to better veterinary care might be simply more dedication by the practitioner. But why is the veterinary profession conducting itself this way? The search for the answers to this question is why I became a veterinarian.

At the time, I took a job at a wildlife center during my under-graduate studies to immerse myself in animal care, and later as an assistant to a mobile equine veterinarian. A pivotal moment in work experience that increased my motivation to pursue a veterinary education was dissection of road kill deer for the wildlife center for the purpose of packaging meat to feed the resident wildlife. The anatomy was fascinating. My family and my wife to be, encouraged me to become a veterinarian. My father was convinced that in order to be successful you had to have a specific science based education that would limit com-petition, and that self sufficiency was the best way to ensure job security. Becoming a Veterinarian fit his criteria and satis-fying him was a requirement if I wanted help paying tuition. Most importantly, both of my parents always led me to believe that their was no limit to what I could accomplish and no shortcuts to the achievement of any career goals. I believed this because I had a successful self made father, and because during the second half of my childhood I reaped rewards from his success and was given some special opportunities that bred confidence and a desire for adventure. I was extensively edu-cated in piano and guitar, spent four summers at sleep away camps including three years as an competing equestrian at Cavalry Camp at the New York Military Academy in Cornwall on the Hudson, NY, completed a month survival course with Southwest Outward Bound and traveled to far away places as a child with my parents including an extensive tour through Europe during the summer of 1972. My father was published and held numerous patents on designs used in air handling equipment including Venturi Scrubbers at the time most com-monly applied in the fertilizer industry. With a successful father as a mentor, and having witnessed and benefited from the fruits of his labor I felt encouraged to follow his example and take on any career challenge of my choosing .

By 1981 at the age of 24 with the promise of family financial aid, I was obsessed with the prospect of becoming a veterinarian, at which time I discovered that entry into these schools was next to impossible and very expensive.

Firstly, my home state of New Jersey did not have one, and there were only 28 schools in the United States and class sizes were limited so that many overqualified applicants were routinely turned away.

I was so dedicated to the pursuing this career that I convinced my high school sweetheart and new wife Mary Ellen who I married in July 1982 to move to Texas in 1983. We settled in El Paso. Across the border in Cd. De Juarez, Chihuahua, Mexico there was a Veterinary School pleased to accept my application immediately. U.S. Schools would have dragged out the application process for possibly years before I would be accepted and matriculating.

This was a great opportunity to get schooled as well as experience the friendly mexican way of life.

Alfonso, a student in my class, became my Mexican brother in the fall of 83, looking out for my best interests across the border. Mary Ellen and I got to know his wife Muryama and family in Satellite Ochenta, a small community out side the city limits of Cd. De Jaurez. I finally had the pleasure of meeting his mother the morning Alfonso and I castrated her 200 lb pig. Afterwards she insisted on feeding us breakfast including home made tortillas. I lived in both worlds divided by a bridge and what appeared to be a brook, but in fact was the Rio Grande River.

I was schooling at the Universidad Autonoma de Cd. Juarez, Veterinaria y Zootecnia with 10 other U.S citizens., studying the veterinary course work in Spanish at the cost of 500.00 per semester. Finding inexpensive tuition removed any financial concerns from our minds. This School would have saved us approximately 100,000 in tuition costs over the duration, if I was to complete my education there.

Historically, U.S. students were successful in this endeavor, and the majority did so as honor students, exempt from final exams. I was also rewarded for my efforts with honor student status, and was exempt from final exams. But, I continued to look outside the United States for an English speaking Veterinary School with U.S. Veterinary Professors, so that learning would be easier, and studies designed to better prepare me for the national board exams. A fellow senior student informed me of Ross University, in St. Kitts, West Indies. They had started a Veterinary College recently as an addition to their Medical Doctor program in Dominica, W.I., and were building a veterinary campus in St. Kitts scheduled to Open in March 1984. This school was staffed almost entirely with U.S. Veterinary School Professors.

I applied, and was accepted and started Veterinary School at Ross University in St. Kitts, West Indies in March 1984. There were just nine students in my class all from the U.S.. It was beginning to feel like this career was truly reachable. Here we were on a Caribbean island pursuing my dream in an academic environment full of U.S. veterinary professors on leave from U.S. veterinary schools. Currently, Ross University, School of Veterinary Medicine is the only American Veterinary Medical Association (AVMA) accredited Veterinary school in the Caribbean.. The only notable difference between education at Ross University and stateside AVMA accredited veterinary schools was the dramatic difference in tuition cost and the lesser calendar time spent to finish the coursework.

At Ross University we saved at least eighty thousand in tuition costs and I finished one year sooner than U.S. students. My first semester tuition was 2,000.

Tuition in those days to complete the graduate veterinary program was approximately 40,000 at Ross University instead of 120,000 at stateside veterinary schools. Before leaving the subject of costs, it is important to note that the current cost of a veterinary education at Ross University has risen to 165,000, causing graduates to carry immense student loans that compromise their standard of living, because veterinary salaries have not increased to offset the cost of a veterinary education. Today, attendance at U.S. veterinary schools can cost as much as 240,000 for the four year graduate program. Factor in the cost of the undergraduate bachelor degree in premedical sciences which must be paid for to qualify for admission to veterinary school and you have a huge financial liability before you pass licensure exams and earn a dollar .

Veterinarians do not earn enough to pay down these huge student loans. According to the AVMA, the average salary for an associate veterinarian in 2009 is only approximately 85,000.

The cost of receiving professional degrees in the U.S. has always been higher than that charged in foreign countries. That factor makes it easier to understand why there are so many foreign doctors practicing in the U.S., assuming the positions that should be occupied by natives of the U.S. that can not afford exorbitant tuition.

Anyway, the coursework at Ross was designed for us to finish four years of education in three years.

Because we did not take typical lengthy vacations between semesters we finished three semesters per year instead of two typically done stateside.

The studies were very demanding, but my thirst for adventure and a solid career were quenched because I had this opportunity to study towards becoming a Veterinarian and live in an English speaking Caribbean culture at the same time. Enjoyable island living and an improved academic environment made studying and taking exams more bearable than in Juarez. The only break in studies and exams would be for four or five days, between semesters when we would venture to neighboring islands for some needed R&R. Great short holidays between semesters were spent mostly with our Caribbean neighbors on St. Martin, St. Barts, Martinique, Guadelupe and Puerto Rico. We worked hard and played hard as it should be. But I did have one major interruption during my academic years. I took a leave of absence to the states for the birth of my first daughter Jillian born Oct. 13,1985.

Now I have a wife, an excellent chance at earning a place in my chosen profession, and a family. From the seat of my motorcycle there was nothing in sight that I thought could stop me from pleasing myself and realizing my American dream. These were three of the most challenging professional years in my life, full of some of my fondest personal memories.

Before leaving this subject, you need to understand that I never applied to any U.S. Veterinary colleges.

There is no record that I was ever denied acceptance. My goal to adventure to a foreign country and be educated in my native tongue was consistent with the student body at Ross University. In fact, the dean gathered a vote from students in attendance and he discovered that almost 100% of the students at Ross preferred to be educated in St, Kitts, instead of in the United States. Ross University was the ultimate answer and destination for the majority of the student body. We were a highly adventurous group of comrades.

Living in the west indian culture was a sensational experience. As in Mexico, the climate and people were warm and welcoming, but the Caribbean waters and english speaking professors were an added bonus. I fondly remember the best years of my marriage to Mary Ellen there as well, because she was my partner, supporting my career dream. Plenty of quality time free of the undesirable distractions that keep two lovers and friends enjoying each others company. What a wonderful place to raise a baby. I remember my wife and I playing with our daughter Jillian outside our mountain home in a kiddie pool with a Cinzano umbrella protecting her young skin from the suns rays. What a warm and safe place for her to play.

We took a picture of her frolicking in our overgrown basil garden and we entered her picture in a Johnson and Johnson photo contest where her photo was given honorable recognition and a prize awarded. Loving each other came so easy, and good friends were made.

In particular our Kittian landlord and his wife Hugh and Margaret Parlee. Almost immediately after moving into their home in Frigate Bay they left for Canada and Scotland leaving us in charge of their home and their dogs Patches and Freddie. Two dogs that gave us countless moments of endearing companionship.

I often close my eyes and return to the island and then fall into a peaceful sleep. Sometimes as I commute on my current motorcycle to work I reminisce about riding in St. Kitts where sugar cane fields and the Caribbean water were at my sides. Sometimes I think I can almost smell the scent of burnt sugar cane fields. The kittian sugar cane farmers would burn the fields after the harvest to return nutrients back to the soil.

I certainly pestered the Parlee's before they decided to rent me their flat high on the mountain overlooking the Caribbean waters to the west of Timothy Hill and the Atlantic on the east of the same to the south of Basseterre, the island capital. Hugh was from Ottawa, Canada and Margaret from Scotland. They treated us like family. Hugh would not take more than 200.00 per month rent including utilities and donated his personal desk to me so I'd have a place to study and looked out for me like a brother.

Margaret was kind to my wife during all the long hours she was alone waiting for her husband to return from school. Margaret had been in charge of a school she designed for elementary grades and Hugh had created a golf course which was in his charge. When we left the Island in June of 1986 after I completed six semesters equivalent to three years of study Hugh insisted on giving us a letter of reference to help us secure living accommodations elsewhere.

The seventh and eighth clinical semesters were to be done in Canada and the U.S..

Mary Ellen, Jillian and I arrived in Fergus, Ontario the Summer of 1986. All our belongings fit in our subcompact vehicle until we finally found a third floor apartment downtown that we could sublet.

Apparently landlords in Fergus will not lease to anyone with children of any age.

For the next four months I worked mostly on large animal farms with Dan Scorgie, veterinarian from Orangeville, Ontario. At the time I wanted to gain experience in areas that were not possible to achieve in suburban America. He was generous with his knowledge and friendly from the onset. We concentrated mostly on beef and dairy farm herd health. Herd health is mostly concerned with increasing the cost efficiency of meat and milk production.

Bovine practice entails a lot of physical labor especially when you are dehorning and maneuvering between uncooperative heavy animals all day for injections and rectal palpations. We finished our requirement there and moved to Stillwater, O.K. Jan 1987, just after we learned that Mary Ellen was pregnant with our second child Abigail.

How wonderful.

I joined clinical rotations for the eighth semester with the seniors at Boren Veterinary Teaching Hospital affiliated with Oklahoma State University, while working in equine practice with Cushing Veterinary Clinic, Cushing, O.K. under Brian McNeal, DVM. and Jerry Woodall, DVM. It was in private Oklahoma practice that I learned the technique for Standing Castration that I used in my CT Equine Practice that I established later. Easterners were not accustomed to performing that procedure on horses in the standing position using sedation and local anesthetic.

The standing castration is preferred by those that have applied it over performing the same procedure on horses in lateral recumbancy, because managing to lay the horse down safely during disassociative anesthetic induction and helping him get up safely after recovery in the field can be a difficult task. More later on disassociative anesthesia. Finally in the late spring I set out to satisfy my last requirement before graduation. I was required to complete an externship of my choice.

At the time my passion was equine reproduction, so I found a great venue in Fort Collins, Colorado.

I was eager to arrive at the Equine Reproduction Lab, affiliated with Colorado State University in the late spring of 1987. Here I was extremely fortunate to work under the amiable supervision of Angus McKinnon. Dr. McKinnon, a published expert in equine theriogenology and native of Australia, was indeed an inspiration to me. I soaked up skills and knowledge like a sponge, on many relevant aspects of equine reproduction including but not limited to mare and stallion breeding management, rectal palpation skills, artificial insemination, semen collection, semen analysis and extenders, and embryo transfer. The time spent with Dr. McKinnon worked wonders for my rectal palpation skills, which helped build my equine practice post graduation.

The end of my formal training and a diploma was now just one move away.

Graduation from Ross University, School of Veterinary Medicine was June 12, 1987 at the United Nations, in NYC.

The next 6 months I took national and state boards and the ECFVG (Educational Commission for Foreign Veterinary Graduates) Exam at Mississippi State University in an effort to qualify for state licensure in the states of my choice. The Educational Commission for Foreign Veterinary Graduates gave a 5 Day Grueling exam at Mississippi State University School of Veterinary Medicine for foreign veterinary graduates in an effort to keep unqualified foreign graduates from practicing in the U.S.. This type of exam is not given to U.S. Veterinary Graduates to check their knowledge and skills otherwise I suspect the AVMA would be sadly disappointed in the results achieved by many unprepared U.S. graduates.

Anyway, I survived all of the grueling exams and chose and received licensure in NY, FL, OH, AZ and CT and took my first paying job as a Mixed Animal Practitioner in April 1988 in CT at a meager yearly salary of 25,600 before taxes. The low salary paid typically to an associate veterinarian made it apparent to me at the onset of my career that the profession and the companion animals we serve did not receive the respect they deserve. Salaries for associate veterinarians are still too small to pay down hefty undergraduate and graduate student loans and be financially secure enough to start a family and qualify for a home mortgage.

The practice was 90% small animal and 10% Equine. I wanted a 100% equine position but I couldn't find a job working in a 100% Equine practice that was within a 2 1/2 drive of my wife's home town in NJ. There just wasn't a high enough horse population in the New York Metropolitan area to support another 100 % equine practitioner. She placed this ridiculous restriction on how I was to choose my first practicing position which caused irrevocable resentment. Now my career direction and development took a back seat to her demands. Her mother ruled her father. I should have known better. "An apple doesn't fall too far from the tree." Aside from choosing a job that I really didn't want to please my wife, it was very difficult to support a family of four on that kind of money even in 1988. I only received the meager sum of 20.00 for every emergency I admitted after hours and holidays. At a minimum, I was assigned a fair portion of the equine cases.

But, hope for a brighter future is very possible when your 31 and your whole career is in front of you.

Somehow you think you'll find a way to please your wife, help animals, even emphasize the species you prefer, and make a comfortable living. After all, you're a young idealistic doctor with a specialized skill with very limited competition. But idealism is soon replaced by realism and disappointment.

I immediately learned that working as an associate for another Veterinarian was not the answer to financial security so I had to quit. I had a condominium mortgage, maintenance fee, two car payments and two children and a wife to support. We had to settle for a small two bedroom, one bath condominium because we could not qualify for a house.

Even with my wife's part time job, we were struggling financially.

So, after 4 months I left and started my own practice in hopes of reaching financial security. This gave me the opportunity to limit my practice to equine medicine and surgery which still continued to be my goal and passion.

My start up supplies fit into a cardboard box on the front seat of my bank owned truck on the doors which read the name of the practice. I was heading toward my first barn call as the owner/

operator of Equine Medical Services in the August 1988 right around the time of my second daughter Abigail's first birthday.

Even If I wanted to practice on dogs and cats, I couldn't afford to open a small animal clinic, and my parents were not interested in offering financial assistance to help me start a CT practice. Remember my father was a self made successful business owner that was hoping I would be the same.

But my small equine practice and my wife's part time job at the newspaper and our tag team baby sitting schedule was not providing sufficient income for a comfortable living because I needed more customers. At the time I unsuccessfully tried to convince my wife to move to Arizona so I could have a better chance to succeed in a full time equine practice.

Az had so many more quarter horses than Ct and could have provided an opportunity for an equine practice to produce a more sizeable income. I took her on a trip in 1989 to Az where we attended an Equine Convention held by the American Association of Equine Practitioners in Phoenix. I took this opportunity to apply for equine associate positions surrounding Phoenix and in Prescott. The latter is where I most preferred to live and practice. I met with many friendly veterinarians but no one could offer even a mixed (large and small) animal position. I needed the financial security of guaranteed salary to make a safe employment transition safely from CT.

I couldn't put my family's financial health at an increased risk. Again, much to my disappointment, my wife did not encourage me at all to pursue this course because it involved moving outside the original 2 1/2 hour drive restriction from her mother's house in N.J.. After returning home to Ct, and as a last ditch effort to sell my case to move out west to be surrounded by quarter horses, without my wife's endorsement, I hired an answering service to answer calls for my own practice that I was proposing in Prescott, Az.. I continually advertised this hypothetical practice to be in the local paper to see how much response I might receive.

Unfortunately, after six months and insufficient inquiries, and no spousal encouragement to look for other salaried equine work elsewhere in more heavily equine populated regions of the country, I decided to abort my dream to become a full time successful equine practitioner.

She was not interested in moving anywhere under any circumstances and divorcing my wife and leaving my two children was out of the question. My dream of operating a practice limited to horses in CT was impossible and over.

So.

All I could do was stay put in Ct, sacrifice my career dream and do anything to at least improve our financial status. Anything meant that I had to include practicing on dogs and cats to make ends meet.

Eventually on barn calls I started to see dogs and cats owned by horse owners and later began to include house calls for dogs and cats. As much as I dearly loved my first wife, the seeds of resentment were planted and the roots of resentment towards my wife began to grow, because I had worked hard to become educated and licensed with the hope of limiting my practice to horses and she in fact discouraged my dream from reaching fruition.

In time this resentment led to separation in 2001 and divorce in 2005 after 23 years of marriage.

As it were, my wife and my small animal clientele dictated what I needed to be to support us. They were interested in what my wife and I referred to as "Cheap Shots" done with a minimal house call exam, which I insisted upon, to save them money.

It was a demeaning experience, from the onset.

Many told me they did not want to pay for my exam and opinion. They claimed they already had a small animal veterinarian and they just wanted vaccinations .

I was guilty of interfering with any relationship they had established with their Small animal Veterinarian, but I did not pretend that I could take care of their pets completely as a mobile practitioner. I strongly encouraged them to keep the relationship at what ever cost with their other stationary veterinarian and or emergency hospital, because the mobile vet is not equipped in the field to service all their needs.. In that context, I took the opportunity to do these low cost vaccinations at their request to keep food on my family's table.

This money making service appeared harmless at the time. This was a way we could ensure that pets owned by cost conscious people received necessary vaccinations. But this method of delivering cheaper vaccinations conflicts with the delivery of quality veterinary care.

Low cost vaccinations evolved ten years later to animals receiving no exams with vaccinations by low balling veterinarians in pet stores. These veterinarians usually do not have an office where they can be reached for traditional veterinary care between pet store visits. This caused these animals receiving vaccinations in pet stores to receive inadequate veterinary attention, thereby decreasing the quality of health they previously had experienced when dogs and cats had to make visits to traditional veterinary offices in order to receive vaccinations. At that venue, routine examinations were performed and necessary treatments were possible and administered.

The commonplace availability of these venues is causing a growing portion of the public to act as if the most important reason we go to a veterinarian, who has gone to great lengths to acquire a great degree of knowledge and skills, is just to get vaccinations and a spay or neuter. Does that imply that the public doesn't believe that dollars should be spent for an exam until there is obvious clinical disease? The "kick in the head" is that these low cost vaccination venues refer to themselves as "wellness centers."

The regular office usually had an opportunity to remedy the shortcomings of the puppy and kitten vaccination providers, i.e. inadequate parasites treatment and control, nondiagnosed and untreated infections and congenital anomalies, etc. when it was time to spay or neuter the pet at the traditional veterinary office, but the increasing popularity of low cost spay and neuter clinics that are not providing complete examinations and treatments have further stopped visits to the traditional veterinary office.

If the spaying and neutering can be done by the low cost outfits, what does that leave the traditional veterinarian? You guessed it.

All the other problems including the ones that could have been prevented with traditional veterinary care and euthanasia.

Before, I sound overly dismal and quick to judge in my outlook, I need to say that there is a minority that truly make an effort for their pets and pursue surgery and treatments at traditional veterinary hospitals and clinics. It is these people that we prefer to attract to my office, because it is these kinds of owners that give us the opportunity to do what we are trained to do while supporting our operation. I contend that they're not just dogs and cats. But, I have entertained the hypothesis that for the majority of clients their pets are "just dogs and cats."

Indifference to conscientious veterinary care is the root of the veterinary health care crisis.

I suppose there is little hope for the veterinary profession and quality animal care if the average pet owner thinks that the traditional Veterinary Clinic or Hospital competes with low cost service centers.

Unfortunately, at this time, many owners either think that we offer the same services at higher costs, or they do not care enough for their dog or cat to justify the additional cost of an exam and further diagnostics and treatments that we suggest. In fact, some owners have requested or tried dictating that I skip the exam because they only want the vaccinations. Why?

Because they have a choice not to pay for an exam with LCP's. The majority is trying to stretch the "almighty buck" at the cost of their animal's care. They can't afford it and/or they have other ways they prefer to spend their money. The great debate is founded here. Does better veterinary care stem from more dedication by the practitioner? Sometimes, but in most cases, I don't think so. Pet owners have to decide what level of care they desire for their pets. Some of the poorest clients choose to bypass low cost providers.

Some of the poorest clients choose to spay neuter and vaccinate their dogs and cats with me at twice the cost, rather than a low cost provider. Why? Because they want their animals better looked after.

They want the exam, the treatments as needed and recommendations on behalf of their pet. However, some of these client are not regular clients because they do not have the financial security. I neutered, vaccinated, heartworm and fecal tested for such a client's dog today and it was a pleasure. They're straight up with me from the moment I meet them. That implies that some of the wealthier owners whom can better afford traditional veterinary services that do not choose to understand the benefits of traditional veterinary care prefer to spend less money for pet health care whether or not they need the savings for another reason or not. Therefore, educating the public to the benefits of selecting a traditional veterinary office is our way to improve animal health care. How does a pet owner get educated to understand the difference between low cost and regular office practice?

It is our responsibility as a recognized authority on the subject to make an effort in this regard.

If I tell an owner that many low cost cat spays and neuters are done with injectible Ketamine and Acepromazine or Tiletamine and Zolazepam without the use of general gas anesthesia causing the animals to feel pain during the surgery, how will owners react?

I have tried to explain this situation without success to some existing and potential new clients whom choose not to believe me, because if this was true then why haven't these operations been shut down?

Simple. It is because "they're just cats and dogs," and these owners want to spend 87.00 to have their cat vaccinated and spayed and if someone "blows the whistle," the price is going to raise dramatically because skilled labor is needed to assist with intubation and to monitor and adjust general gas anesthesia.

Even the veterinarians involved in these low cost procedures are at fault for allowing this method to exist.

Doesn't the Hippocratic oath state that we as Veterinarians are to eliminate animal suffering or words to that affect? You bet it does. And that goes for healthy as well as terminally ill patients.

The unacceptable comeback for not increasing the public's awareness to this fact is that if the price escalates for altering cats then many cats won't be spayed and the cat population will get even larger.

On closer examination of this situation, since I began practicing in the 1980's, gas anesthesia on intubated animals rather than injectible restraint has always been a safer, humane, and affordable method to employ to get these cat and dogs spayed. When I started practicing in the 1980's, Methoxyflurance and

Halothane patents were expired and they were the inexpensive gas or inhalent anesthetics of the day and should have been used as the general anesthesic on all these low cost procedures instead of Ketamine or Tiletamine injectible chemical restraint. Isoflurane was adopted by the the end of the decade but its cost was considerably more.

But, Isoflurane was safer for the animals, because the Veterinarian gained more immediate control over the depth of anesthesia in the patients maintained on Isoflurane. For this reason I chose Isoflurane and discontinued use of Halothane even though the expense of Isoflourane was considerably more. Because the welfare of the animal instead of the cost should be the foremost consideration. The cost in 1990 for 100 ml. of isoflurane was approximately 68.00.

Today , because the isoflurane patent has expired, a 250 ml. bottle of the same is approximately 20.00.

Now it is possible to provide an even safer economical gas anesthesia for cat spays and neuters. But for just a few dollars savings in product and two hours skilled labor costs, injectible chemical restraint with Ketamine and Acepromazine and Tiletamine and Zolazepam are still inappropriately used causing discomfort to the cats during these procedures because they're not fully anesthetized. The truth needs be known.

Ketamine and Tiletamine are disassociate Anesthetics that do not produce general anesthesia and therefore do not produce visceral analgesia and do not remove the cranial nerve swallowing reflexes to permit intubation, therefore they should not be used for any spays or neuters.. Without visceral analgesia means that the female senses and reacts to the procedure performed on her abdominal reproductive contents and or the male reacts to castrations performed on his reproductive anatomy . Furthermore, in any case, without intubation, the airway is compromised and aspiration of saliva and stomach contents into the lungs is a possibility.

The dissociative "anesthetic state" produced does not provide general anesthesia or fit into the conventional classification of stages of anesthesia, but instead produces a state of unconsciousness that appears to block only some sensory impulses sent to the brain. In addition to cranial and visceral nerves, spinal reflexes such as the pedal reflex remain active as well. These unconscious animals respond to these procedures by kicking their legs as well as contracting their bowels making the surgical procedure more of a risk to the patient.

These active visceral, cranial and spinal reflexes are not appropriate during surgery. Conventional general gas anesthesia removes or sufficiently reduces these undesirable reflexes during surgery.

Owners must be obligated to pay for skilled labor and general gas anesthetic so that a non painful humane procedure is done at a price that is realistic to help defray the costs of operating a conscientious veterinary clinic or hospital.

Many unaware owners think we are overcharging for anesthesia. The fact is that LCP's are avoiding the necessary labor and gas costs to perform these procedures on intubated animals receiving gas anesthesia as it should be.

The cost of a spay or neuter done at my office and other traditional providers is continually challenged by pet owners who falsely believe that they can get the equivalent procedure done by a LCP for less than half the fee. I think it is unusual to pay half as much and expect the same results. Under the circumstances I would think a cat spay and vaccinations done by a LCP at the ridiculous price of 87.00 should be questioned, if the going rate at a regular office is approximately 250.00.

On the contrary. I am put on the defense. Many pet owners only think in the moment and are too easily persuaded by the dollar sign. As a result we have lost a large part of the vaccination and spay and neuter business to low ball operators that do not and will not provide the same conscientious humane approach to veterinary care now or later. Why should owners defend these LCP's?

Where are these Low Cost Providers when your pet needs everyday veterinary treatment for a condition?

Not available, not equipped and with no intention to help you.

Mrs. B brought in her 8 week old male intact (MIT) Shih Tsu, because the "hospital" she had a prepaid care contract with for vaccinations and neuter was not able to perform surgery to remove a dermoid cyst from his cornea. This is a hair producing mass that is found on the temporal region of the cornea.

I gave her a quote to excise it and did so as soon as her husband cashed out funds from his 401K. Apparently, the LCP "hospital" that operates in the back of a pet store is unable to perform this procedure and they will not give her a refund to help pay for this surgery. I will take this opportunity to point out that unless you are able to overnight patients that you should not refer to yourself as a "hospital."

This "hospital" refers to itself as one deliberately to mislead the public to attract as much easy money as possible. What other reasons would they have for doing this? If people knew upfront that they could not overnight patients or perform procedures that require more surgical expertise they would loose a large portion of their audience and income.

When they call themselves a hospital they mislead pet owners including Mrs. B, by giving the impression that they are capable of performing most surgical procedures and handling hospital cases that require overnight care. If asked by their clients about cases that obviate overnight hospitalization or that require surgical expertise above the typical spay, neuter, simpler dental and small superficial cutaneous mass removals, they will volunteer that they have a relationship with local veterinarians for that purpose.

If that was truly the case, why wasn't Mrs. B referred to a veterinarian that they are affiliated with to perform this surgery. Simple. Because they do not have such a relationship! This shortcoming in their level of service should be obvious to pet owners.

Hello.

Veterinary clinics such as this one that lease space from the pet stores can only operate when the pet store is open. Adhering to the pet store hours of operation means that they could never provide overnight hospitalization when the pet stores are closed for business since everyone has to vacate when the store is locked up for the night. How could this misconception be prevented to protect the consumer?

A government law should be put in place to prevent these veterinarians from misleading the public in this manner. There needs to be a law to define when the word hospital is permitted in a practice title to protect pets and their owners. This law will assist in the survival of traditional veterinary hospitals that provide overnight hospital care and more surgical expertise benefitting the delivery of higher quality veterinary care as it should be, and eliminate the poor conduct of veterinarians in this scenario.

The owner returned with the dog and I did the surgery to remove the dermoid cyst from the cornea. Because she had prepaid for the neuter with the pseudo hospital, I could not neuter her dog at the same time which would have been a medical decision in the best interests of the dog.

Why is that you should ask?

Because the LCP refused to refund her money and the owner was only willing to pay the cost of the eye surgery. Neutering the dog at the same time with one anesthetic exposure instead of two is a safer choice for the dog but this concern is not a priority to the veterinarian at this LCP, or even a priority to the owner. Their priorities are dollar driven.

It is important to note that if this dog had went to a traditional hospital which is more equipped and more able to perform a wider array of surgical procedures, that this dog would have been neutered at the same time as it should be at a savings to the owner.

Did she save money and make the best choice for the health care of her pet at this national "Hospital"?

No.

Meanwhile my practice has lost approximately one third of its yearly income, and our community has suffered a loss in higher quality veterinary care over the past few years because of these imposters.

Before closing this subject I need to add another detail.

I job interviewed with this national "hospital" so I could tell them that they shouldn't call themselves hospitals inside pet stores to solicite their reaction. It is my impression after that meeting that they do not care that they are deceiving the public because they are quite comfortable telling clients "they work with other local veterinarians if the need arises" You and I know by now that this is not the case in my experience and that they should be providing the services the public expects.

They do not want the responsibility for any complicated care. How does this fact rest with you? Do you want to be turned away by this "hospital" when there is a medical crisis with your pet, especially when time is of the essence.

Absolutely not.

They have put the pet, the pet owner and the livelihood of the traditional veterinarian, who delivers more valuable services, in a vulnerable position.

Try calling up a traditional practitioner you do not know, tell him "Rover" had two rounds of vaccinations, heartworm testing and neuter done at a low cost service center and that you would like to get "Rover" in immediately today because he's not feeling well. Do you now expect this veterinarian to come to your aid immediately and whole heartedly. Of course you do. The Lord teaches us to do on to others and we would want done on to ourselves…

The saddest part of the story is that the animal ultimately may not get the medical attention it needs if the veterinarian is disinterested in prioritizing this patient and he conceivably put his loyal clients ahead of the new comer. The typical excuse provided by the owner for this situation was that he or she didn't have enough money to come to a "Regular Veterinarian."

What is a "Regular Veterinarian"? Is there a separate more advanced degree given to "Regular Veterinarian." Absolutely not. Does "Regular Vet" means they will pay more for the same services? Yes, because operating a regular office entails maintaining the expansive inventory and available skilled personnel to provide many types of medications and appropriate treatments at a moments notice. An owner wants and demands this sort of service and he needs to understand that this comes at a higher price.

Unbenounced to many owners, low cost centers do not acknowledge many diseases and are not equipped for a diversity of treatment types especially at a moments notice. Furthermore, paying the price demanded is not negotiable. Why do some people think that we welcome price haggling at our offices?

How many times have I heard when an owner calls for a procedure price quote for a cat that the cat is just a stray. They think
that the 'Regular Veterinarian" can be convinced to lower their
prices for this poor little homeless creature. The part they conveniently leave out is they are adopting the cat into their home
just as soon as the reduced bill is paid, and thereafter we will no
longer be referring to "Precious" as a stray. The cost of animal
care is not on a sliding scale. Products and labor are at fixed
prices that only rise not decrease over time. It doesn't matter if
we operate or provide medication for one, three or twenty animals, the cost is the same for each patient with the same approximate weight.

Price breaks are offered at the generosity of the office under only
special circumstances. For example, one of my client's dog needs
a kart in order to get around since his back injury. These karts
will cost at least 400.00, and usually I offer a treatment discount
to owners for these patients, because I need the owner to purchase one of these costly carts, otherwise treatment results are
compromised and their pet's chances for survival is reduced.
This cart will provide external immobilization, expedite convalescence and alleviate a great degree of discomfort.

Certain products and medications are difficult to purchase by
some folks whom truly are trying their best to help their pet. By
their actions, it's not difficult to eventually discern whom these
people are.

Unfortunately Ms. M after four months still didn't purchase the
cart in spite of my generosity at the payment counter. Treatment
that includes a cart expedites the recovery of the patient because
the back is kept more immobilized, making it possible to
shorten the length of steroid treatment for the spinal nerves. I
prefer to reduce the length of steroid treatment, because in
many cases long term steroid treatment with prednisone may
cause unwanted side effects including cushings disease, gastrointestinal hemorrhage, hepatitis and even shock causing

death. I warned this owner about these side effects and finally insisted before the third refill that I would not give her any more prednisone unless she purchased and started using the cart. At that time she again promised that she would purchase it that day and that she had enough prednisone to last another week and a half so that we could keep her dog on the medication while we waited to receive the cart due to arrive by carrier in three days. Two hours later I got a phone call from a receptionist at another veterinarian's office 20 miles away that wanted the records sent because Ms. M had an appointment the next day. I explained the situation to the receptionist and she said she would definitely tell the veterinarian to call me the following morning before her appointment to discuss the situation. I never heard from this veterinarian. It's probable that she got prednisone from the other veterinarian and never bought the cart. I suspect that eventually this dog passed away from aggravated back disease and iatrogenically induced hepatits and or hemorrhagic gastroenteritis.

Here is good example of how owners play veterinarians against each other to save money and get what they want at the expense of sound veterinary healthcare. Veterinarian aware of these practices, need to remember to prioritize the animals needs first, rather than their desire to fatten their "bank accounts." But in some cases, just the cost of medication can be the cause of poor treatment results.

Animal drug companies need to keep their prices reasonable as a first priority, so that the veterinary cash customer can afford and benefit by their products. Let's remember there is no government health care program yet to assist in the payment for their products as in human health care.

The bigger animal drug companies, whom support costly sales presentations and expense accounts are frequently charging more than the market will bear for the products they're pushing. Currently, I can't afford to carry all of them, or compete with the low cost vaccination and spay/neuter centers. Prior to the mid

90's , before low cost service centers, there was more interaction with pet owners. A large portion of our income was generated spaying, neutering, heartworm testing and administering vaccinations at a fair price. This lost revenue to low cost vaccination providers helped support my practice to the extent that I could better afford to purchase more expensive medications, and better afford the opportunity to provide more costly treatments, at a lesser profit to improve overall animal health care. Therefore, it is important to note that "Low balling veterinarians," whom cause a reductions in visits from a significant portion of our clients and our income are contributing with the high cost of pharmaceuticals and biologicals as important reasons why we're unable to deliver higher priced advanced care that the animals need.

I will take this opportunity to mention that the environments where low cost services are provided are typically substandard. These settings are presenting a poor image of the veterinary profession. I typically hear how owners have dropped their cats off in carriers in a parking lot to be spayed by and vaccinated on a truck. What kind of respect is the public to have for our advanced services if any of us are willing to work under such deplorable conditions.

Furthermore, there is no doctor-client-patient-bond (DCPB), and the owner is completely ignorant to what is needed or recommended for their pets care. Dogs receiving surgery at low cost spay and neuter centers on occasion have post op complications and the surgeons can not be reached for follow up care.

A gentleman who was doing sign work for me, told me about his dog who received a low cost spay and experienced post op complications. He could not reach the low cost surgeon, and brought his dog to an all night emergency clinic where the dog died. His family was gravely disappointed after this event. These types of irresponsible low cost services send a terrible message to the community about veterinarians.

When there is substandard conditions and no doctor-client-ani-
mal bond this is what can happen. Another factor that has
decreased this necessary DCPB is the purchasing of on-line pet
prescriptions.

"Hi this is On Line Pet Rx's, Mrs. R. would like a refill of
Cyclosporine Ophthalmic ointment, 25 mg. Rimadyl, and Iver-
heart Plus. Do you authorize her prescription refills?" What
they should ask is: Do you take responsibility for any complications that may result after we supply the medication?
Strangely, the courts rule in favor of the clients demanding that
we o.k. the refill unless there's a reason why we shouldn't.

But, how can we ascertain the reason if the owner denies us the
opportunity for a current physical exam and a chance to study
the current history. When the on line agent identified the owner
to be Ms R, I called her to discuss her dogs history.

The dog's history alerted me to require another physical exam.
As it turned out she would have re-ordered Rimadyl which was
not the drug of choice. The dog is now suffering predomi-
nantly with a neuromuscular back condition and needed to
start prednisone and stop Rimadyl. In addition I recommended a cart which was never purchased to expedite the dogs
convalescence. Typically, every week I am bombarded with
requests from third party on line pharmacies to refill my clients
with medication. Sometimes, without any facts it apparent to
me they've surfed the company's web site and picked out what
they think they need, then asked these agents to call and ask
for my authorization in hopes of avoiding the cost of my services at the risk of their pet's health.

Fortunately, at this date in most cases the requests for on line
prescription refills are for Heartworm disease prevention medication. But, the last one was for a dog I hadn't seen in almost
3 years. This particular client Mr. L., has a dog who has stayed
current on Heartworm preventative. I gave him the courtesy of
a 12 month refill last year from my office without his yearly

exam when it was 2 years since a visit, with the advice to bring the dog for a check up. One year later, now after three years he'd like me to authorize another on-line corp. to refill the same medication. It's apparent that his interest in a relationship with me to care for his dog has ceased to exist. I refused the request by the supply co. and he did not schedule an appointment for an exam as I again requested.

If I gave them permission to refill his request, then the dog would not be obligated to visit with any veterinarian until his rabies vaccination expired, because only veterinarians are authorized to administer rabies vaccinations. I can only hope for the dog's sake that he doesn't hire a Low Cost Vaccinator (LCV) in which case the dog will not be examined for health.

Does the breakdown in the DCPB occur when the owner thinks we're money hungry?

On the contrary, it's the owners of these animals that are truly prioritizing money as their primary concern.

They do not want to pay for a health exam, our advice and our inventory because they question the value of our opinion. Our selling price for these products are similar to those found on line. Surely, they must understand that selling these prescriptions help support our practice. Therefore, asking me to allow a third party to refill their prescriptions certainly won't nurture my relationship with them. So, what else could be a reason why they choose to avoid their pet's veterinary care provider.

Control? Are these people control freaks? Are they afraid that they will be exploited because we will coerce them into purchasing unnecessary products and services if they were to bring "Rover" in for a yearly check up? In the exam room, when I mention a surgery that would improve the quality of their pets life, .i.e. surgery to correct Third Eyelid Gland Prolapse and Entropion (inward folding eyelids) I feel I better insist that the surgery is not a requirement. Why? Because if I don't, they might think I'm money hungry. But, I can loose their respect if I don't mention that the lacrimal discharge in either case will continue unless the surgery is done.

Choosing to ignore the problem or giving them an Ophthalmic ointment to temporarily relieve irritation which will only cease to work when the medication is stopped will mislead them to think I do not understand the condition. Only approximately 10% of the entropion and 60% of the Third Eyelid gland prolapse cases will ever be surgically corrected by any practitioner. Apparently, I do more prolapsed third eyelid gland surgery because that disease is more difficult for the owner to live with. The pets level of difficulty is a secondary concern.

The damage to the cornea by entropion that is not surgically corrected can be extensive over the life of a dog. Speaking of the cornea, we diagnose a considerable amount of dry eye or Kerratoconjuctivitis Sicca (KCS). We start the Cyclosporine Ophthalmic drops to increase tear production by the third eyelid and accessory tear glands and after two to three months the cornea is adequately hydrated.. But only 10-20% of cases continue to pick up the drops to maintain corneal health, at the cost of about 20.00/month..

Maintenance dosing is just one drop in each eye once daily.

Is the labor of permanently medicating the dog and/or the expense to much for the owner to justify; How can they look at their dog 's dry pasty opacifying corneas and witness the blindness that ensues without the use of the ophthalmic drops?

After 30 to 60 days of cyclosporine ophthalmic drops the corneas are moist as they should be, and they will stay that way preventing this cause of blindness if the owner can just once per day put a drop in the affected eye. I suppose the labor and/or expense is the reason why less than 20% of Crystaluria cases in dogs and cats are maintained as they should be on overpriced prescription diets to stop disease.

Presciption diets are used with this urinary tract disease to keep the quantity of crystals in the urine to subclinical levels. Mr. W. tells me the prescription diet for his dog for triple phosphate crystals is too expensive and he is considering euthanasia, because without prescription diet his dog has accidents and eventually hematuria (bloody urine).

We tended to his dogs Triple Phos. Crystals trouble with great success for four months until we never saw him again, ten months ago. "The treatment was a success but we lost the Client."

In theory a practice should be built on treatment successes, especially when it's done so at a very competitive price. Another client that required the same diet, known as Mr. M wanted me join the barter exchange or sell him larger volumes of this prescription diet to reduce the price on more than one occasion.

I do not get a quantity discount on this product and I'm not interested in bartering so again I lost that client over high priced prescription diet. I provided him with almost ten years of faithful service. Since then I have eliminated over priced prescription diets from my practice and substituted them with lower cost manufactured and compounded prescriptions to increase owner compliance and retention, because the cost of prescription diets are not reimbursed by private veterinary insurance companies. But the cost of routine medications, which can be reimbursed by private insurance has caused noncompliance too, because many owners can not afford private insurance or even inexpensive services or medications.

I just finished an appointment with a cat who I prescribed antibiotic and digestive enzyme powder for diarrhea secondary to what I suspect may be Pancreatic Disease. She couldn't afford hospitalization or lab. work to confirm the diagnosis. So, rather than do nothing I advised her based on the exam and history to try some treatment for Pancreatitis. The owner said she could only buy only one oz of the enzyme powder from me, and that she could get the antibiotic suspension cheaper from her M.D. at 13.00.

I told her that I needed to dispense all medications as needed so that I can ensure product accuracy and quality before I would take any responsibility for the treatment of her cat. She agreed.

Why must I have to be put through this kind of an ordeal on a regular basis? In her case, I later learned from her coworker, that she has more than twenty cats kept in a trailer. Would she have been able to accept the medication and my prices if she didn't have too many cats to care for? I don't know her well enough to predict the answer to his question. But, after 25 years in private practice, I have reasoned that the dollar sign is a bigger concern than the wear and tear on our relationship. In her case, I believe she exposed her weak financial status, instead of the excessive number of cats she has trouble caring for, as her best argument to convince me to try to help her cat at a price she could afford.

Obviously, there should be laws and enforcement to limit the amount of family pets allowed per household to prevent this type of situation. There is not a devious plot to exploit veterinary services in this case. This woman is acting out of desperation to help her cat. Each owner cares for their pet(s) at a personal and financial level that they are comfortable with. Unfortunately, too many pet owners willing to care for their pets can not even afford to take care of one pet when they need the most help.

Recently, a 5y neutered indoor only cat presented lethargic, mildly febrile, tender abdomen, mucous membrane color normal and 7% dehydrated. According to the owner he has had projectile vomition for one week already.

She fed him and gave him water since this began because she did not call for any advice. Apparently she hoped she would not have to consult with me to save money. After an exam, I informed her that the cat needed to be hospitalized to survive and receive all medications thru his I.V. catheter including sufficient fluids to help re-hydrate him and assist his body to correct his acid-base imbalance. I told her I would send out cost conscious rudimentary blood tests to assist in the diagnosis and to better assess his organ health status and have more information to share with her about her cat tomorrow. I kindly asked her for a four hundred dollar deposit so that I could cover my start up expenses. She responded telling me that she could only raise two hundred dollars, but if she called her mother who is living off her deceased husband's life insurance policy that she may be able to raise another two hundred. I charged her for an exam and asked her to bring back the cat back just as soon as she could arrange payment for the deposit. She never came back with her cat that day for the hospital care the cat required in order to survive. Simply put, this cat required hospital care and she could not afford to take care of her only cat. I suspect, she will battle with the consequences and her conscience after this is over.

If I can battle with mine as you have learned in this book, I suppose there are pet owners whom will do the same. Because owners have very limited funds to allocate to the veterinary care of their pets, I have become defensive about adding important products on to an invoice that are not a requirement on the day of treatment.

A typical scenario can be that an owner will come in for a yearly check up and overdue vaccination for multiple pets and quickly state that they only have a couple of hundred dollars but they definitely need a popular flea tick medication before they leave. I typically state before beginning that it's the check up and vaccinations or the product. Then they act overwhelmed by the cost of these products and wait for my sympathy and cooperation to provide all the above. All I can do to stay in business is first state that we take all forms of credit cards which many say is out of the question, and then do the check up leaving out higher cost Lymes vaccination, do not refill heartworm Rx, break up the boxes of flea/tick and give one applicator per dog instead of sell the packages of three or six doses as provided and the bill in this case added up to only 230.00. Even though I have made every effort to limit their cost, I discovered they were short, and we had to wait for her husband to come down and pay the small balance or hold two flea/tick applicators for her to pick up later. Meanwhile there was an office full of clients observing this situation with similar financial predicaments. This scenario reinforces the opinion by some that we as "regular veterinarians" are charging too much for regular care which motivates them to use a LCP, where they can have complete control over the cost of services and not have to undergo any embarrassment at the time of payment. But I suspect there is another reason why owners are selecting low cost substandard services.

Owners are electing inferior veterinary care because they prefer to feel satisfied after a visit for veterinary care. When an owner visits my office for me to examine their pet, with good intentions to do my job to the best of my ability, I discuss and recommend any diagnostic tests or treatments in an effort to provide the best care I can for their pet. After all the exam, consultation, and available treatment options and recommendations is what defines the difference between traditional veterinarians and low cost veterinarians at vaccination venues. Then we discuss the cost of these procedures and the owner frequently does not elect the procedures because of their financial limitations, causing some of them to feel like they are irresponsible pet owners. In affect, pointing out their shortcomings as guardians can cause them to feel inadequate about how they care for their pet and their experience at traditional veterinary offices. This can cause some pet owners to steer away from traditional veterinary facilities towards low cost vaccination clinics so their not later reminded of conditions that they have not attended to. Ignorance to their pet's health status, after visits to low cost vaccination centers where exams and recommendations are non existent or incomplete, is bliss.

They leave there feeling content about what they have done for their pets. We can not remove this lower cost temptation for pet owners by competing with these low cost providers, because keeping the costs down further on the invoice to keep the client compromises the quality of our services and animal health care.

Dropping costs further requires eliminating some necessary vaccinations, heartworm prevention medication as well as eliminating recommended diagnostic tests and treatments to alleviate disease.

Ms. LB just asked me to quote price for a canine spay. If I start telling her that the dog is overdue for an exam, vaccinations, heartworm medications, etc. in addition to the spay at additional cost, I will loose the business to a LCP, who doesn't care. Why is that?

Because LCP's do not take any responsibility for the dog's overall healthcare, they will just spay the dog as the owner requested and ignore other medical and surgical concerns. But, aren't all veterinarians ultimately the ones that are take the responsibility for these animals?

If push came to shove the answer is yes. But, since many pet owners are now dictating who, how and where services are performed and for how much it is difficult to hold any Veterinarian accountable. Is the fault really with the veterinarian for a long term roundworm and ear mite infestation that caused the long term diarrhea and eventual vomiting and aural hematoma that could have been prevented.

In fact, on closer analysis, the fault should be with the owner. Often I request a stool sample and the owner conveniently forgets to bring in the sample. Often I prescribe treatments that are not carried out. Chronic otitis, in some cases accompanied by repeated mycotic aural hematomas with the same patient are not unusual, because these owners are saving money by choosing not to purchase the long term maintenance ear care product I recommend and sell.

Noncompliance with medication recommendations to save money cause chronic ear disease and chronic urinary tract disease. In the case of crystal caused urinary tract disease, obstruction and even death can occur in some cases. There are many more examples I could offer where noncompliance to save money causes many unnecessary chronic diseases, but these two simple examples should be sufficient to make the point. The cost of veterinary care has become an obsession with consequences for pet owners.

I just got a telephone call from a lady who asked me how much to spay the cat. I said, if that is all I'm concerned with and you want me to ignore any others needs, which is not the way I work? Then she said "yes." Then I told her the price and she said " Thank You" and "Goodbye." She didn't ask what else her love one might require and invite a discussion. Why? Because, some pet owners have lost respect for the profession. The loss of respect for the profession has caused these owners to disregard our advice or take matters into their own hands.

Fourteen months ago, I made Mrs. G aware of the severity of the peridontal disease in her cats mouth very apparent to her. In fact the swelling and foul odor from the mouth especially in the area that included an abscessed tricuspid molar was very obvious. She did not want to spend the money to correct the problem.

Since then she has chosen not to discuss this fact until I noticed it again when she presented the cat for routine vacci-nations this year. This year with most of the teeth in this cats mouth loosened as a result of advanced periodontal disease, she would still have disregarded the problem if I had not made her a charitable offer she couldn't refuse. This deal which included General anesthesia, eight extractions, injectible antibiotic, long acting anti-inflammatory injection, seven days of dispensed antibiotic and a Rabies booster and overnight hospital care was done for 300.00.

Wow. How low does the price have to be for owners to elect treatment?

She still complained that she thought the fee was pricey.

This cat should have had routine pre-op. blood work run including Feline Leukemia and Feline Aids testing to try to better understand why this 5 year old cat had such advanced periodontal disease. Furthermore the cat has conjunctivitis. But I had to disregard the findings of the eye examination and diagnosis, because the budget was already too low and my first concern was alleviate the oral discomfort this cat was experiencing.

The depressed value of the dollar should not leave anyone in sticker shock at 300.00 for this level of professional service. So, I am inclined to believe that this owner does not truly respect our services.

Because If she did respect traditional veterinary services which includes advice, why isn't she appreciative of my concern and gracious about my efforts on her cat's behalf?

The popular option to seek services with LCP's, and choose less care is a root to the veterinary healthcare crisis. This causes owners to make uninformed choices for the healthcare of their pet. As a result, every week we receive paperwork consisting of incompletes. Incomplete vaccinations, dogs not on heartworm prevention, animals not spayed or neutered, not on antiseizure or thyroid medication, etc.. Just like a report card when the student drops out of course. These pet owners like dropping out of class, have dropped out of traditional veterinary health care as it should be.

Some owners driven to cut traditional veterinary costs want what they want and that's all there is to it.

These types of owners will call and ask for a price quote on just "all" the vaccinations. "All" the vaccinations to them means Distemper and Rabies. In Connecticut, all dogs because they step outdoors, should also receive Lymes vaccination and be on Heartworm preventative.

It's come to the point where if I insist on this when trying to schedule the appointment, I will loose the opportunity to meet the owner and the chance to deliver the advise and care the animal deserves. If this type of client makes it to my exam room they often are opposed to following my instructions to the letter because they think they're "calling the shots." They want to be in control like they are when they visit LCP's.. These "Find the Lowest Price for the service they want Hunters " have acclimated to picking and choosing their services at LCP locations. I can not help this type of transformed pet owner, and I prefer not to because they usually do not follow all my instructions, not reaching the results I predict and their outcomes may reflect unjustly on my reputation. It's the old clients that I've seen year after year where I've earned their respect, that I choose to help that are more likely to comply with my requests and follow thru on my treatments, as well as the clients that are victims of LCP's that ignored and/or mistreated their animals, and pet owners that have not been exposed to the LCP that make the best clients.

Another source of difficult clients to help may be those who have received services from a Mobile Veterinarian. Especially the mobile veterinarian, who claims he can perform heroics if needed on the owner's kitchen table. Mrs. A came in the other night and told me the mobile vet is back and how he used to come to her house. She said that he told her he would perform surgery on her pets on her kitchen table if they needed it. I asked her if it was necessary to clear the dishes first? How ridiculous.

Veterinarians like this have contributed with the LCP's to making sure our image as professionals is degraded to the point where maybe the owners feel that the time has come that they better, instead of the veterinarians, start making safe choices for their pets. Maintaining a low operating overhead is a common reason for many mobile veterinarians, but encouraging and rationalizing surgery on the kitchen table instead of a clean and equipped operating room stocked with adequate supplies and ready personnel is inappropriate. It sends a message that we think practicing under compromised conditions is acceptable by the veterinary community.

What a pitiful professional image this creates for any observers. This poor image contributes to the disrespect towards veterinarians and ultimately towards the disinterest in traditional veterinary care. Some green mobile Veterinarians after they've created enough client base and income never build an office to perform procedures. I have seen invoices from career mobile veterinarians that list prices compatible with high overhead offices. This high profit earned by these mobile vets. should after sufficient time be put toward building or even leasing an office to perform certain procedures in a more professional and suitable environment. But the profits are not used for the purpose of improving the image and care provided by some of these veterinarians.

When I started in 1988 I didn't have the funds to open a downtown office. As already mentioned, I strictly ran a lower overhead equine and small animal (dogs and cats) mobile clinic for four years until I built a house at which time I was able to create an office in my walk out basement to better care for my small animal patients. The mobile clinic and my dream as an equine practitioner lasted only six years, from 1988 until 1994 under the name of Equine Medical Services.

The care I provided towards horses remains as the favorite years of my professional life where I was always eager to treat reproductive, lameness and colic cases.. I sold my dream to stay put and please my wife. My only hope left was to attain financial security for my family of six. I gradually went from 100%

Equine in 1988 to 100% dogs and cats in 1994. I was tired of struggling to support us and made the difficult choice to grow the more lucrative small animal portion of the practice and phase out any equine clientele.

My wife and I received appointments with dogs and cats in the humble four room home office I constructed to improve our image and services from 1992 until 1998. It had a separate entrance to a waiting room, and included an exam room, surgery room and lab and cage room. Meanwhile in order to support ourselves and build a larger small animal clientele I was humiliated as a veterinarian to have to work in pet stores throughout the state for three years to increase our exposure, which added to the resentment I carried towards my wife.

For this reason we named the practice: Statewide Veterinary Clinics. My wife joined me and we took the practice on the road, even while she was pregnant with our daughter Caroline in times of severe winter weather, and we provided limited conscientious outpatient veterinary care at as many as ten pet stores throughout CT visited monthly or bimonthly. During these times I was blessed with a third daughter Sara two months after moving into that house in 1992 and a fourth daughter Caroline in 1995. Her efforts were admirable, but we were in this predicament because of her refusal to allow my career choice. That would have involved a move west where I could find full-time employment in equine practice.

This was long before vaccination clinics were ever seen in pet stores. Unlike today, if I determined that a dog or cat I saw at the pet store needed further care I would schedule them at my home office between visits, because my goal was to build a practice that provided complete conscientious veterinary services.

It wasn't the career choice or office of my dreams, but as soon as I could afford to I opened a humble office in the city in 1998 to better care for my patients and provide privacy for my family of six.

Caring for my daughters gave me more incentive to live with the humiliation of part time "pet store practice."

It was difficult to pay all the bills to support the house, the practice and the children, but we always tried to represent ourselves as professionals. I wasn't proud of the environments we had to work in and we knew our limitations, and did not hesitate to recommend specialists at another venue if the animal would be better served. By the millenium our income had finally risen significantly so that we were taking vacations, had already built an in ground swimming pool, bought a time share in Jamaica, leased several expensive cars, etc. but the resentment I held toward my wife could not be forgotten.

It didn't matter how many toys we bought or vacations we took, the marriage was crumbling.

Finally, I met someone that would happily help me achieve my current aspirations. At the time I wanted to create a second home and second practice in Florida. My first wife Mary Ellen did not even want a second home in Florida as a compromise. Her comment was "move down there by yourself and when it's all set up and running in five years, give me a call." It was more of the same kind of resistance from Mary Ellen.

LuAnn, my second wife to be in November 2006, stepped into the picture after I left my first wife, twelve years after the Az experience in 2001.

She was a breath of fresh air. She eagerly helped me make a home and practice in Florida.

Unfortunately, I lost all my Ct home equity to my ex-wife, absorbed the enormous legal fees and was held completely responsible for all family expenses and debt in the divorce in 2005. They let me keep ownership of my Ct office so I could pay for child support, generous alimony, and college tuition.

The financial security I had finally acquired was sacrificed and the Florida practice and lifestyle that I wanted for LuAnn and I became compromised. Now I had sacrificed my equine career and financial security to my first wife Mary Ellen.

LuAnn and I couldn't make ends meet in Florida, so that the Florida dream did not happen either, even after an attempt at three different small office addresses over a six year period. It was too difficult to pay the increased obligatory expenses in the divorce "agreement."

LuAnn was so eager to please me in the first two Florida practices while they each failed. The Ct practice which I maintained to help pay for our Florida life, and the loss of my share of the home equity to my ex-wife and alimony payments after the divorce left me in too weak a position to support and hold on to our dream of full time residence in Florida.

By 2005, after the closure of the second FL office I was convinced that we both needed to move back to CT full time in order to survive financially. By this time I had a loan on FL property and a building contract for our future home which needed to be paid for. LuAnn worked with me in Ct from 2006-2007, to help us save money and generate more income. But the financial obligations put forth by the divorce settlement and the economic recession that later emerged in the winter of 2008 caused too much financial stress on our relationship, so I decided to minimize expenses and make one last attempt with an office in Florida in the winter of 2008. This last time was the only time I attempted a full time work and personal life in Florida. I went so far as to close my Ct office and Ct house to reduce expenses so that my effort in Florida could not be compromised by any financial obligations in Ct. We personally packed up two moving trucks with a car in tow and moved backed to Florida in January 2008 with hope of never returning to CT again. By this time, LuAnn and I chose not to work together in my third Florida Office that opened in March 2008 to spare our relationship any further unnecessary stress. On the bright side, we were able to live in our Florida home full time for at least six months in 2008. It was completed in April 2007. For a brief period in 2008 we had a taste of what our dream would have been like if we succeeded.

But, I could see the imminent failure of this third office immediately and closed it in the summer of 2008 to conserve any savings we had left.

With no other viable job choices, I immediately set out to reopen my CT practice in hopes of regaining any lost clients, and to hold on to our Florida home. We were both so disappointed that we had to leave Florida and live full time in CT that it almost ruined our marriage.

I finally changed the name of my CT practice to Statewide Veterinary LLC in July 2008 when I moved back to CT to a larger office for two main reasons. Firstly, because I had confined myself to one city for already 10 years, and secondly because the word clinics has become associated with low cost limited services. I refuse to be considered a LCP with limited irresponsible veterinary services.

The public will not respect our profession if any of us represent or conduct ourselves in an unprofessional manner in an inadequate environment producing substandard results. We have an obligation not an option, to represent ourselves to the public in the most professional manner, and that includes discussing all the diagnostic and treatment options available. For example, if the dog needs a fiber optic exam of his rectum and you do not have a fiber optic scope we must send the patient to a hospital that has one. But having a state of the art office doesn't mean you will always have the chance to practice at that level .

Providing the highest level of care is not possible when the owner elects not to pursue a more costly definitive diagnosis and subsequent treatment Rather than do nothing, I may reluctantly agree to conservative treatment. I explain up front that the results are less likely to be successful when we are denied use of advanced diagnostic tools to confirm a specific diagnosis, and advanced treatments to improve the outcome.

Seven days ago a seven month intact male domestic long hair (DLH) cat presented. The owner's boyfriend wouldn't allow the cat in the house because he wasn't neutered yet. The smell of cat urine is strong and offensive on intact male cats so he felt justified to leave this cat outside at all times at whatever risk until after the cat was neutered. Thus far the cat has not been examined by a Veterinarian, and he has lived steadily outside for five months under his "care."

He presented weak, inappetant, third eyelids raised and other systemic neurological deficits, bilateral nasal discharge, afebrile, 5% dehydrated with an orange tinged chemical on his feet and abdomen. The boyfriend indicated that he attempted to wash this chemical off him yesterday. The owner had to borrow 400.00 from her father in order for us to admit him to our hospital. Blood chemistries, CBC, urine analysis, FeLv, FIV, testing did not reveal anything noteworthy except a mild leukocytosis. A toxicology screen for pesticides, herbicides, and ethylene glycol (Antifreeze) and possibly a spinal fluid tap and analysis should have been run immediately on this cat, but the owner's father cooperation to pay for all these tests was questionable.

When a patient is very sick on presentation it is difficult for an owner to take the financial risk of spending his money on diagnostic tests and treatments without any evidence of a good prognosis.

My costs on a Cerebral Spinal Fluid (CSF) fluid analysis and the toxicology testing without labor costs is at least 300.00. Adding this to the above tests already run would have put us deep in the red before I began any treatment to stabilize the cat.

With the given financial limitations, the chance to find a definitive diagnosis in not possible. Instead, the owner limited financial support, limits my plan to the basic blood work already noted, an I.V. catheter, and fluids and medications needed in attempt to help the cat process the chemicals and/or infection.

I need to point out that giving us sufficient funds to spend on any diagnostic tests that are necessary to confirm a diagnosis helps us to better understand how to recognize, diagnose and treat diseases and therefore become better Practitioners.

The small four hundred dollar deposit for this cat was consumed five days ago and I am making every attempt to manage this cat conservatively to give him a chance to survive. Three days ago I neutered and vaccinated him against Rabies so that the owner will let him in the house for at home treatments. I practice in hopes of payment to cover expenses and make a comfortable living. I need to point out that if the cat expires before final payment, that it will be difficult to collect any further payment and we may loose money in an effort to help this cat.

Because of typically reduced payment for services when an animal passes away, cases with a poorer prognosis constantly threaten my practice's solvency. We should not have to operate our practices in fear of loosing money in an effort to succeed with our more challenging cases.

Typically, when a cat or dog is admitted to the hospital the first course of action is to obtain blood and urine samples to determine a treatment plan. Many of these animals have not eaten or drank sufficiently in days causing dehydration. In these cases, elevations will occur in serum urea (BUN) creatinine and phosphorous which could look like a kidney disease and cause a premature inaccurate diagnosis of reneal (kidney) impairment. If the kidney is truly involved these elevations over the normal range will persist for 7 or more days. If they are elevated because of simple dehydration they will reduce to the normal range in 2-3 days with I.V. fluid rehydration. It is for this reason that hospital time is required to arrive at a more accurate diagnosis and prognosis.

Owners want a diagnosis as fast as possible to reduce their investment, but I must emphasize that hospital time is required to reach a diagnosis and prognosis.

Recently a 16y S/F DMH cat present with this history. Elevations in BUN, Creatinine, and phosphorous were found. The owner was told from another veterinarian that she was suffering from kidney disease and that the prognosis was grave. This conclusion was reached after a simple office exam and a single serum chemistry profile.

I hospitalized the cat and these values were found in the normal range after my second serum chemistry profile taken after 3 days. On the second day of hospitalization the cat was repeatedly observed seizuring. Anti-seizure medications were started and she did not respond favorably. Meanwhile, I.V. Fluids with dextrose kept her glucose levels within normal range.

I was able to ascertain that she had a neurological disorder instead of kidney disease after three days. If she had an acute reversible kidney disease she would have had a fairly good prognosis, but she had a neurological disease non responsive to anti-seizure medication after two days of therapy. Her prognosis was grave due to a neurological disorder, not a kidney ailment. In too many instances, owners do not have the money to pay for 4 days hospitalization, diagnostic tests and treatments to determine an accurate diagnosis and prognosis. Instead these cats and dogs are euthanized to spare expense making it impossible to practice quality veterinary medicine. Veterinarians are apprehensive about taking on these cases because they are a gamble.

The gamble has to do with receiving payment. How do you feel about paying for services if your cat or dog is dead after 4-5 of hospitalization, diagnostic and treatment costs. In these cases, we are accustomed to reducing the bill and not recovering payments for our services, lab fees and products, which can cripple us financially. It is for this reason that many veterinarians will not take on these challenging cases. How would MD's react if they ran the risk of insufficient payment from all their patients whom did not respond favorably to treatment.

Fortunately, the previous chemically poisoned DLH cat is now eating and taking oral medications twice daily, but only because my technician helps him to do so. This cat stayed in our hospital for one week. On the sixth day, I was able to convince the owner to permit me to repeat the basic blood work to check for delayed evidence of kidney and liver damage. The blood work was completely normal, and I released the cat on the seventh day to keep the costs down. Relying on the owner for his early convalescent care is risky, because of the owner and boyfriend's questionable nurturing capabilities. Too many owners will not even spend enough for treatment at this lower level of expertise.

Recently I had two cases of acute renal impairment presented due to ingestion of toxic materials. In the first case the owner suspected paint chips were the cause and in the second floor cleaner. Either way, these cases required longer hospital care then most can afford. The first case stayed with me one week and the other case nine days until the blood creatinine, urea and phosphorous levels started to drop down significantly enough so that they could resume eating and drinking without vomiting. On average, if I flush their bodies daily with I.V. fluids for 3-4 days then Subcutaneous fluids adding dextrose for nutrition for seven to ten days, I can then send them home stable enough to resume normal lives. Because the bill is too costly for most owners to contend with, I offer a significant degree of charity to make treatment possible at my hospital, otherwise these patients would be euthanized by others.

Again, many hospitals will not absorb the cost of this treatment and these animals are instead euthanized to spare costs for the owner and prevent non profit services by the hospital. In good conscience, I elect to absorb these costs and save these animals lives, because my first thought is to save their lives then try to figure out how to make it as affordable as possible. I chose to be a sole proprietorship so I can have the luxury of this decision whenever necessary. I do not need the agreement of partners or corporate executives to save these dogs and cats.

Notice, I used the word luxury.

Yes, I make multiple trips myself to the office to save labor costs, close off the hospital room and run a space heater to save on utility costs to make this possible. My low overhead, and personal sacrifice makes these treatments a possibility, even though many owners believe I am charging too much.

Any hospital and/or surgical cases, over $1,000.00 can raise suspicions, even though the fees are very reasonable for the services and products consumed.

Recently, I palpated a mass in a cats abdomen and to spare costs took the cat with the owner's consent immediately into surgery. I.V. fluids, CBC, chemistries, celiotomy, bowel resection and closure, daily fluids with dextrose and antibiotics for three days hospitalization and dispensed antibiotic caused a bill to reach 1,374.00. Radiographs were omitted to save the owner money since the findings on palpation were sufficient to justify surgery. The owner saved more money by denying a biopsy of the mass attached to the jejunum and mesentery and cytology of the abdominal effusion. I discouraged omitting the biopsy and cytology reports because I need them to render a prognosis. But again the "almighty buck rules". As it turned out the owner was suspicious and not grateful for the services I performed to save her cats life. In fact she demanded I give her the biopsy in formalin and the tube of abdominal effusion so that she could bring it to a third part to verify my work. How about that… But I am not that surprised.

Ten days later my technician told me she removed a bag from the outside door handle from my office. The bag contained the biopsy jar and the tube of abdominal effusion. No written comment was enclosed. Apparently she never surrendered the specimens for analysis to another office, because if she did she would not have been able to return the samples to us. Such drama.

She was upset with me from the onset when I gave her an estimate of at least 1200.00 to treat her cat, instead of pleased at what I can accomplished for a very reasonable fee.

If these services were performed by my local competitors whom have more overhead, the price would surely have been at least double after three days hospitalization.

A more reasonable price is still too much to pay. It doesn't matter how skilled the services and how great the value because the price is still unaffordable. It is difficult for me to go a good job at a remarkably low price and take on sticker shock complaints. Conservative care is the treatment of choice for many pet owners.

Mrs. SB is expected in the office momentarily to drop off her cat for individual cremation. She wasn't even willing to pay for the lab work that I suggested at the time of her visit two days ago. The cost she is paying for individual cremation exceeds the cost of the blood work I requested when I administered conservative nonspecific outpatient treatment for her cat. I took the opportunity to ask her if she was satisfied with the unsuccessful results of the non specific conservative less costly treatment her cat received that I did not prefer. She said yes, because she thought the cat was too weak to undergo the diagnostic procedures and any intensive treatments that may have been necessary for her to survive. She believed that any money spent on the lab work or radiographs would have been wasted. I then asked her why I wasn't alerted to the cats recent health status before she became moribund. She said she didn't bring the cat in sooner because she thought the cat was dying from end stage urinary disease and that all she could do to help the cat was to make sure she ate her prescription diet.

Another treatable condition or hospital care to improve her cats chance of survival was inconceivable to her.

But in some cases, costly diagnostics and hospital care can reveal diseases that are not treatable. How do you feel about spending 1,000 to find out that there is nothing you can do to save your pet? But without a diagnosis, a poor or grave prognosis and/or irreversible suffering, I will not euthanize an animal.

I can not put a pet to sleep at any age who is not suffering or even one who is in discomfort without a diagnosis and prognosis, just because an owner doesn't want to seek a diagnosis for financial or any other reason.

I'm frequently confronted to euthanize many aged animals I've never met as if by command. When I refuse their command what happens to these animals?

I suppose they call around until they find a veterinarian who will take their orders or the animals are neglected. and continue to suffer. Many owners believe that it's their right to end their pets life without medical advice.

Many years ago a horse owner wanted me to put her healthy horse, who was in my care for years, to sleep just because she was moving to Florida. She didn't want the horse to make the trip and she didn't want the horse to have a new owner.

This notion that we can be commanded to euthanize an animal means that those holding this opinion believe that veterinary treatments including euthanasia are a choice that is made completely at the discretion of the animal owner for their animal that is either healthy or diseased.

It is my opinion that if we act on these commands by owners to euthanize animals that we will by our actions make this notion seem correct.

The public needs to be made aware that this conduct toward animals is illegal and immoral. We as veterinarians need to defend animals rights in these situations, otherwise we will loose our purpose, which is to safeguard the health of the animals. We can only do this by insisting that respect and care is given to the creatures in our care.

But how do we defend these animals and insist on appropriate care when the owners are not cooperative ?

Firmly refusing the command as I did to put the healthy horse down is the first step.

Mrs. P just dropped her cat off for blood work. She thinks the cats is all done. I told her without a diagnosis that I could not consider euthanasia. I did blood work, administered fluids and a long acting antibiotic injection with outpatient instructions to with hold food for 48 hrs.

As it turned out CBC and Chemistries revealed a hemolytic disease. This thirsty small appetite 12 year old cat who is continuing to loose weight with formed stools might be easily mistaken for having renal insufficiency if lab work was not done. If that were true, euthanasia might be a reasonable course of action. The blood revealed no abnormal findings except an increased total bilirubin, low hemoglobin, low red cell count and low T4. I called her and suggested following a treatment for Hemobartonella (Mycoplasma) and Autoimmune Hemolytic Disease (AIHD). She agreed to try. If I was the type of Veterinarian to simply follow her orders, I would have euthanized this cat three days ago. Better still if I was the kind of Veterinarian that was tired of insisting that owners pay for even rudimentary lab tests, the cat would be in my freezer today. I am pleased to tell you that I hospitalized the cat and started treatment yesterday for hemolytic disease including those caused by Mycoplasma and AIHD and the cat is still with us today.

He actually took a few mouthfuls of dry food today. I will keep this cat with me until I feel he can take care of himself, except for daily meds the owner will have to administer to maintain or finish a course of treatment.

I am fond of Mrs. P and her family, and am anxious to please them. I have known them for 15 years.

Folks like Ms. W mentioned before who couldn't even afford conservative treatments I can't help.

In fact, at the risk of seeming heartless, I should refuse administering conservative treatments (those done without any tests taken), because operating under these compromised conditions yields much poorer results, which reflects badly on my reputation and the profession. The best I can do to give the animal a good chance of a successful treatment and support my practice is not to underestimate the willingness of the owner to pursue a diagnosis and treatment. That means I should not hastily sum up a clients capability to comply with costs and other challenges to pursue and treat their pet.

A new client we will call Mr. P telephoned me two days ago and asked how much for a physical exam to examine his dog's leg that has been swollen for weeks. He said he could raise the 45.00, but any more would be difficult because he was only receiving disability compensation. I agreed to see him promptly.

After the exam I had determined that the 7 year old neutered Pit Bull had pulled a Right Hock ligament severely enough to cause insertion site swelling and sensitivity. I recommended radiographs, a cast to immobilized the joint and Calcium supplementation. The owner agreed to pay the estimate of charges and to do the procedure asap.

The dog was admitted and discharged yesterday after receiving all the procedures recommended and the balance paid in full. I could have assumed that since it was difficult for him to raise the 45.00 for the exam, that he would not be able to afford basic diagnostics and treatment.

It's Thursday morning Feb. 18, the phone just rang and I answered. The question was and you guessed it "I'm calling to inquire about euthanasia, how much to do it for my cat" My reply was have I ever seen the cat before? She replied "no." I then answered that I can not euthanize her cat unless the diagnosis justifies that action. She then hung up on me as I was about to try to build up hope by saying that there is a cat in my hospital now that is responding to treatment that would have been put down 4 days ago if I was to simply have put the cat to sleep without insisting on a diagnosis first. Again, it is apparent that this owner thinks they have complete say so about this subject regardless of my opinion as veterinarian.

Just before that, I got a phone call from Mr. P about his cat that is in my hospital undergoing treatment for Hemolytic disease. Instead of asking me how his cat is doing, he commanded that tomorrow is the cat's last day, and then I need to euthanize him.

I told him that the cat ate some dry food yesterday and appears to making some progress. If I release this cat before he is well enough they will bring him to another Veterinarian who will not be given the opportunity to help him.

Mr. P picked up the cat after a 7 day stay in our hospital. As discussed the cat's blood work for the most part was normal. I learned that while with me he ate in a manner that was typical for him throughout his lifetime. I sent him home with thyroid supplement and prednisone suspension, and to encourage treatment cooperation and no hard feelings, I charged half price for the care of the cat. Thirty six hours later without even the courtesy of a telephone call from Mr. or Mrs. P, I received a fax from an emergency clinic where the cat was euthanized at the owners command. I suspect the two of them couldn't deal with any treatment requirements, and as she already told me she "didn't want to look at him anymore." Even though I had a telephone call with Mrs. P the night of the cats discharge when she told me that she would give him another week. She did not. Remember, she's the one that wanted euthanasia from the get go.

I suspected this might happen if I released the cat before sufficient recovery, but after a week it was not affordable to keep the cat any longer under my care.

These clients adamantly believe that it is their decision regardless of prognosis to end the life of their pet, and that I should respond to their command. According to the fax I received, their was no new lab work or other evidence that the cat's condition had deteriorated in the thirty six hours since I discharged him to warrant euthanasia.

Diseases that require a extended convalescence such as Mr. P's cat often do not get the chance to survive

Recently, after a very long relationship with this client I was asked to send their records to another veterinary office for future "care" of her other animals. I gladly accommodated their request, because I choose not to work for pet owners that do not care to endure long term treatments at home.

But, aside from emotion, the cost and the labor to administer medication daily can be too much to encumber for many owners. After all, he is just a cat? Why do I keep talking about euthanasia? Because every day I spend a large portion of my time supporting health care as alternative to euthanasia. I was trained to practice medicine and surgery to keep our pets alive and healthy as a first choice. Hospital care costs to treat pets is unpopular with clients especially if more than three days are required. The cost is considered by some to be overwhelming especially when a guarantee for survival can not be given.

I require hospitalization when an owner inquires such as Mrs. R. about care for their pet who has been vomiting for days, because a successful outcome depends on medication and fluids given by injection only.

Mrs. R said she couldn't afford the $400.00 deposit and hospital time to care for her one yr. male pit bull. She was hoping there was something I could do less costly for her dog as an outpatient. Months later, I saw her with a different dog. I learned that the one yr. old male pit bull had died at home after lower cost outpatient "care" by a competitor.

He did blood work and sent her home with oral medication which served no fruitful purpose except to produce a bill. To get paid, he did what she wanted. Meanwhile, he mislead her into thinking the dog was dying of kidney failure after one initial blood test to "wiggle" himself out of the difficult situation he had gotten himself into. He should know that without hospitalization this dog would die. Claiming there was kidney failure was done to shield him from blame for the dog's death.

As previously discussed, the compromised kidney needs at least three days of I.V. fluid therapy and other injectable treatments to excrete backed up metabolic waste. Again, it is commonplace that dehydrated dogs and cats have initial blood work indicative of potentially irreversible renal disease. Only after 3-10 days of I.V. fluid treatments can reversible elevated readings for Blood Urea Nitrogen (BUN), Creatinine, and Phosphorous have sufficient time to fall into the normal range, vomiting to cease, and the patient be discharged. None of these patients should be sent home until they are stable. This period of treatment must be performed and blood work repeated before determining the prognosis of the kidneys.

This vet. should have told her the dog required hospitalization to administer I.V. fluids and other treatments by injection. Two professional opinions in agreement should have convinced Mrs.

R to admit her dog for treatment, in which case he could have survived after 3-10 days of hospital care. It's disturbing that she blames herself for her dog's death, because she did not follow my recommendation.

She said to me, "I killed him. I should have let you take care of him. If this ever happens again, I will do whatever you say. I will get the money somehow". I told her the dog died because of the other poor advice she received from the other veterinarian.

It should be criminal for a veterinarian to render a diagnosis and prognosis prematurely, and not insist on the best treatment plan for a patient.

Money is the cause of death of this dog. In this case I place most of the blame on the veterinarian. He wasn't honest with the owner. His conduct caused unfair treatment to the dog and an emotional scar to the owner.

Frequently, hospitalization is required because a pet has to have medications delivered by injection because the animal will vomit if any oral fluid, food or medications administered. This more cost intensive hospital stay could be avoided in non-vomiting cases if the owner could pay strict attention to our home care instructions on administering medication.   But many owners think they can determine better what they need to do. Against my advice, some owners will not pill their pet with just water and insist that they can only accomplish pilling if the pill is rolled up in a treat. Non compliance here often causes the dog to start vomiting.

Once vomiting begins so does dehydration, acid base imbalance, lethargy and eventually starvation.

Furthermore, once vomiting has started no oral medication or fluids can be given and the pet frequently has to be hospitalized to survive because the only way to receive treatments is by needle or I.V.. Ms. B brought her 11 y Black Lab to see me16 days ago. She presented with swollen retropharyngeal lymph nodes, fever of 105.6, enormous tonsillar hypertrophy and anorexia. I took blood for a CBC and Chemistries, administered I.V. Fluids, antibiotics and released her the same day with home care instructions to keep costs down at the owners request. Incidentally the dog has various lameness conditions responsive to carprofen. The discharge instructions were large doses of antibiotic for the infection and carprofen for fever reduction and lameness. I asked her to call me in about 5 days to let me know if she felt a reduction in lymph node swelling so that I could determine if I needed to continue or change the antibiotic therapy.

Instead she called me 10 days later after the dog had been vomiting for a few days I learned that she was giving the medication with table food against my advice. She decided cheeses were o.k..

At the time of that telephone conversation, I instructed her to not give any food, water or medication for 48 hrs. and administer antibiotic pills after that only if the vomiting ceased for the same 48 hour period. But vomiting continued because she continued to give her water against my instructions There is a good chance that giving the cheeses repeatedly, after our first appointment, with all the carprofen and antibioitic medication caused the emesis to begin. She did mention that the dog was eating, drinking and acting much more normally and the lymph node swelling did reduce somewhat on the medication during the first week of treatment. The CBC and super chemistries did not indicate any remarkable changes except for the dramatically high WBC count (55,000) and elevated bands, indicating a severe infection. A simple outpatient case of infectious respiratory disease has turned into a case that requires hospitalization because outpatient instructions were not followed.

Because the owner can't afford the cost of keeping the dog in the hospital so that we can make sure nothing is given to her orally and to treat the dog by injections, euthanasia of a dog for what was a simple respiratory infection is now a topic of discussion. Often, I have to compromise the preferred method of treatment or the dog or cat will not have a chance to survive. Today, Saturday, to avoid the cost of recommended hospital care for this vomiting dog, I gave the dog 1.5 liters of LRS S.Q. and two antibiotic injections one of which has a two day action and again gave the instructions of no per os. until we speak Monday. I reduced costs by administering subcutaneous fluids instead of I.V. fluids because the antibiotic I prefer to give is expensive to give orally for 4-6 weeks to a 90 lb.dog. I hope vomiting ceases and we can start it Monday night or Tuesday. Further delay in oral antibiotic treatment will decrease the chances of the dogs survival for monetary and medical reasons.

In the end, because the owner could not afford hospital care and couldn't follow outpatient instructions the patient did not survive as an outpatient at a higher cost than anticipated.

This dog passed away because she did not have the opportunity for an extended hospital stay as initially recommended, because the cost to do so was prohibitive to the owner. Electing lesser preferred treatment protocols and poor compliance causes unnecessary disease, costs, and death. Non compliance with instructions can lead to hospitalization for what could have been very manageable conditions. Government financial assistance is needed to help cover hospitalization costs to stop these unecessary deaths.

Recently an elderly couple considering euthanasia presented their 18y A/M Black LabX who was having difficulty ambulating, urinating and defacating on himself, with advanced cataracts for a diagnostic work up and hospitalization after my insistence. Fortunately, the owner left a 400.00 deposit to cover some start up expenses, but she did not hesitate to inform me the funds were to be taken from her savings to pay yearly taxes. The history from my records revealed that they had been non-compliant with my instructions, which were to continue an anti-inflammatory for arthritis and eye medication to clarify his lens that I dispensed to them five months ago, which turned out to be the only reason why the dog needed this hospital stay. We drew blood immediately checked his blood glucose, and sent out samples for general chemistries and cell body counts (CBC), administered I.V. Fluids and kept their hospital bill down to 624.00 after two days treatments in an effort to give this dog a chance at survival.

Since he appeared dizzy, we needed to rule out diabetes immediately. Fortunately, his blood glucose was normal as well as the remainder of his lab results.

Currently, the public should know that if the dog was hyperglycemic and diabetic, that we could not successfully treat him because our last source of insulin that was effective in dogs and cats, namely, Bovine Protamine Zinc insulin is not available. It is pathetic that insulin effective to maintain life in diabetic dogs and cats has never been consistently available since I started practice in the 1980's.

Therefore, many canine and feline diabetics have died unnecessarily because the production of suitable product by the pharmaceutical industry has not been given serious attention. Thus far, typically only a handful of skilled pharmacists have been our only unreliable source from time to time. If government insurance for dogs and cats was available as a source of reliable income for the pharmaceutical industry as it is for humans, dog and cat insulin would have been continually mass produced and marketed many years ago.

We as veterinarians can always successfully treat diabetic dogs and cats if effective insulin is always available, and the owner can afford sufficient hospital costs to stabilize glucose levels prior to the patient's release. But until then, any owner who had a pet that needed effective insulin when it was not available will surely believe that a diabetic pet has a poor or even grave prognosis. Furthermore, this situation may even cause many pet owners to unjustly believe that perhaps we as veterinarians are not as competent as human physicians, when in fact we are not to blame. In any event, I believe that government financial assistance to help make veterinary prescriptions available and affordable will increase compliance and improve animal health care which will result in eliminating some costly hospital stays.

Mr. M just telephoned me about his cat who I diagnosed 3 years ago with FUS (Feline Urological Syndrome) which is essentially urinary tract disease caused by triple phosphate crystals in the bladder and urethra. The cat has since been presented unlike all other cases of this sort at least twice per year with repeated bouts of this disease. The reason is because his wife prefers to feed him food other than the costly prescription diets I have advocated. She recently brought the cat in again. The cat has been completely incontinent for two weeks and as a result they been confining him to the half bathroom in their home. Because they have not complied with my instructions the animal has suffered unnecessarily. Again I keep the costs to a minimum by dispensing medication, not insisting on hospital care, so treatment is affordable enough to try. Owners will push for euthanasia on these very treatable cases if I do not assist them with lower outpatient or hospital costs to remedy their poor performance as care givers.

These sorts of situations have worn my patience thin over the years.

Remember Mrs. B who I previously mentioned at the start of the book whose husband was out work for 15 months? She brought in her new puppy to see me for her first visit yesterday. She didn't labor over the decision to pay for a new puppy.

She took the free advice of her breeder and brought her to a "wellness center," aka LCP for first vaccinations. She only asked for a four way vaccine at the free advice of her breeder, which did not include Leptospirosis. No stool examination, no Lyme vaccination, no heartworm prevention medication dispensed, and worst of all no physical examination or sound advice was given, as typical at the "wellness center." To save purchasers money, breeders frequently recommend LCP's as if they're doing their buyers a favor. On the contrary, in fact, since LCP veterinarians do not offer advice, sending them to "wellness centers" causes unnecessary diseases to occur and the public's ignorance to persist about veterinary health care. Pick your own fruit at the farm to save money is a different matter than pick your own vaccinations and treatments. Pet owners often act on free veterinary advice by non veterinarians, i.e. breeders and pet store associates which is often just as harmful to the pet as it is to their pocketbook.

Usually, whenever unskilled free advice is given it's not worth anything. I can ask the check out person at the grocery store how to care for my water heater. Often with good intention, she'll give me free advice.

But it is not helpful. A plumber will be content to offer valuable advice on water heater care when you have paid for his services. Breeders and pet supply stores give a lot of free non useful and even potentially harmful veterinary advice to their customers. Excellent examples are Glucosamine supplement to alleviate arthritis, Dental treats for plaque and tartar control that work poorly and often cause gingivitis, over the counter diets for dementia, and the control of urinary tract disease that do not perform as labeled. Frequently labels will say these products are vet. recommended.

Which vet recommended these products? There is no name of the vet provided on the packaging. I certainly do not recommend these pet stores products to treat these diseases.

Why go to the vet for advice? All the pet store products are vet recommended. You don't need to pay for professional advice, because the pet store already has the products we endorse.

Nonsense!

The public has been brainwashed by pet store product merchandising and false TV, periodical and package advertising. Laws should be designed to require a veterinarians name and contact information be provided with any product that he or she recommends. This rule would stop many misconceptions.

When the owner and pet finally shows up in my exam room with overdue dental extractions and an urgent need for major tartar and plaque removal, is when the owner is enlightened. They may argue that they used dental treats to control dental disease that are vet recommended. My comeback is that I do not endorse these products. I suggest that they save the money that they would spend on dental treats for a thorough veterinary exam and competent cleaning always done under anesthesia. Groomers whom charge for teeth cleaning are also guilty of misleading the public. Their service is so inadequate that it should not be attempted & illegal.

In order for adequate patient cooperation to perform a thorough exam and cleaning of the dental arcades the dog or cat has to be anesthetized. This fact should be obvious to pet owners, since they will struggle with anyone whom tries to hold their mouth open just for a glimpse.

Pet owners are wasting money on dental treats and groomer teeth cleanings that should have been spent for services by a veterinarian. Laws should be implemented to restrict dental work to be done only by licensed veterinarians. In equine practice I had to contend with the "Equine Dentist".. He or she pretends to provide complete equine dental care.

I found that their service was restricted to a partial float in most instances. Because horses have continually erupting teeth, floating must be done with a rasp to smooth the outer upper and inner lower edges of molars. Sharper unfloated edges compromise the grinding efficiency of these molars causing decreased food consumption and assimilation, resulting in weight loss and reduced performance.

"Equine Dentists" are not veterinarian or licensed doctors of any kind and therefore are not able to administer tranquilizers or anesthesia to perform any dental procedures. For this reason, it should be just as obvious to horse owners that they can only provide very limited services on a cooperative animal. Exams are not done and the lower teeth do not get floated by these imposters because the practitioner has to hold the tongue out of the way to complete these tasks. Very few horses will cooperate with tongue restraint and the floats in motion in their mouth without a tranquilizer. Furthermore, to examine the rear teeth I would install a McPherson speculum in the horse's mouth and crank it open. I never had a horse that could tolerate the McPherson speculum without at least a tranquilizer. So here we have it.

The equine Dentist does incomplete exams and floats and gets away with it. I would point out the shortcomings of the equine dentist to clients, but they wouldn't believe me. People are under the impression that there are consumer protection laws already in affect to prevent this sort of deception. Not true.

A law should be enacted to limit any animal dentistry to licensed veterinarians. The Dept Of Consumer Protection should stop these imposters. The public needs to be guided by laws to steer away from these imposters to ensure their pets receive the appropriate advice and treatment. Have you ever consistently received good free advice from anyone outside the specific field of expertise? No.

In fact, the free advice to select LCP's veterinarians whom do not offer advice, or accepting free advice from non professionals frequently cause owners to end up paying more for "regular" veterinary health care because treatments and recommendations were not given to pets and owners respectively in a timely manner. For example if the roundworm infestation was diagnosed at 8 weeks old by a "regular" veterinarian, instead of a food allergy by the pet supply store sales rep, dewormer with a treatment plan to end the lifecycle, would have been dispensed, instead of a lamb and rice dog food, so that emaciation, vomiting, diarrhea would not have ensued requiring costly hospitalization for I.V. treatments including fluid therapy when the puppy is presented weeks to months later gravely ill at the "regular veterinarian's" office.

The general public has defined these LCP Veterinarians as not "Regular Veterinarians." If a woman telephones my office and says she already has a regular veterinarian, that means she's is under the impression that I could be a LCP with limited services and a discounted rate, I immediately set her straight that I do not resemble a LCP in any way and proceed to define the difference.

Exposing the LCP's for what they really are is one step in the direction towards creating a more healthy conscience concerning how we care for animals. As already noted we can start with stopping the use of dissociative anesthesia used for low cost spays and neuters, and stopping the disregard for timely fecal flotations and lifecycle treatments to better stop intestinal parasite lifecycles from persisting. LCP's deworm pets without first performing fecal flotations and then ask for a stool sample prematurely on the next visit leading sometimes to false negative readings on the next visit causing chronic intestinal parasite infestations to exist until they are seriously ill and seek "regular veterinary" attention. But in order to improve the delivery of veterinary services we must change the way people think about the animals with whom we share the planet.

I recently saw the movie "The Misfits" with Clark Gable, Marilyn Monroe, Montgomery Cliff and Eli Wallack where in the end they released the wild horses they had captured because Marilyn Monroe did not approve of how they were treating these horse that were to be killed and there carcasses used for dog food. Many men are not as sensitive as women to animal welfare.

For example, this past Saturday a man and women presented a cat after regular office hours that I haven't seen in five years because of decreased stool production and flatulence. I remarked that it was a good move for them to reach me before I left the office, otherwise they would have incurred more costly emergency service rates elsewhere typically incurred on the weekend. Her husband standing behind his wife and I standing over the exam table quickly commented that he wouldn't subject himself to those rates and instead would choose the bullet for the cat. His wife was quiet. But she and I know that the only reason that the cat was in my office for attention was because she insisted. Because men respond to women, as in the movie is the reason why many animals get better treated. Probably, 75% of all appointments kept are held by females, unless euthanasia is on their minds.

Just now the telephone rang and I spoke to Ms. R. She indicated that her dog died yesterday at 3:20 PM.

She was a spayed female Lhasa admitted last week with history of vomiting and lethargy.

But, even though she cares, because of her limited finances, the dog was only hospitalized for the day to save her hospitalization costs against my better judgment, instead of the 3-5 days that is typically recommended to make sure the dog is stabilized after a treatment plan is formulated and executed.

Blood work was run and radiographs were taken, I.V. fluids and injectables were administered before discharge with explicit instructions for no food or water for 36 hours. Meanwhile, there was ample time to receive results from blood work due back in less than 12 hours. At the time of discharge, the dog was alert and responsive. I spoke to her the following day and advised her that the dog had Pancreatitis and Diabetes Mellitus. At that time I learned that she was letting him take water against my instructions which caused further vomition. Due to the severity of the dogs condition, I advised her to withold food and water again. I did not hear from her again until later in the week at which time the dog was in a more severely compromised condition. Because she had no funds, she did not call me. She still could not raise any more money to hospitalize the dog. She convinced herself that she was doing everything that she could do until the dog died.

I never had the chance to begin insulin therapy and stabilize the pancreatitis, because she could not afford the hospital time and treatments necessary to stabilize the dog.

I repeat, these dogs need to be hospitalized so that instructions can be carried out to the letter, and stabilization is possible but many owners can not afford it so our results are compromised. I strongly feel this dog could have survived this incident if she could have paid for hospital care. What a pity…

In these cases I have three choices: Free Treatment, Free Euthanasia or escort them to the door in hopes that they can raise money for treatment. Option three is the most realistic choice. I finally received a follow up telephone call with Ms. R on Monday when she informed me the dog had passed on Sunday. She indicated that she had the dog cremated thru a hospital almost an hour away. I asked her why she went to such a great length to find that place. She said that she was under the impression that I did not provide that service. What a convenient excuse to not communicate with me. Most likely she conveniently presented the dog dead or moribund to an emergency Veterinarian on Sunday, who euthanized the dog and had the dog cremated. On Sundays, emergency veterinarians usually work at a disadvantage because they have difficulty receiving records from other offices on their day off. I never got a message with a request for medical records concerning this patient from the office she went to on Sunday.

The woman doesn't truly understand that if adequate funds were provided I would have hospitalized her dog and probably would have saved her. Her concept of medical and surgical care as a means of helping her dog ceased to exist after the 500.00 she borrowed, eventhough the dog had initially showed encouraging signs of improvement and had treatable diseases.

What we need is national government regulated and funded medical insurance for animals just like we have for people. Medicare and Medicaid were established in 1965 for that purpose. If we didn't have Medicare for aged and Medicaid for the underprivileged many more humans would suffer today as the companion animals do today. The public expects veterinarians to just take on the expense for the needy without sufficient reimbursement, or perform euthanasia as a remedy to this situation.

Would any MD today feel comfortable with our predicament.

It's time the Government stepped in as they have for humans to help our family pets, namely dogs and cats.. Many pets are not treated or even put to sleep when they're suffering, because owners can't or won't spend sufficient money on veterinary care.

Treatments are ignored or results are compromised because of a limited budget.

Many of these animals could have been saved and go on to sustain productive lives for years.

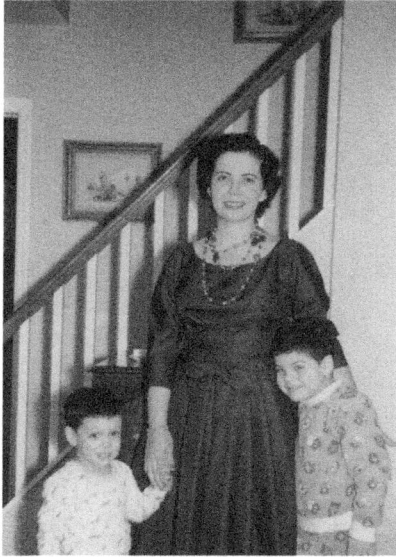

Mom holding my hand with my brother circa 1959

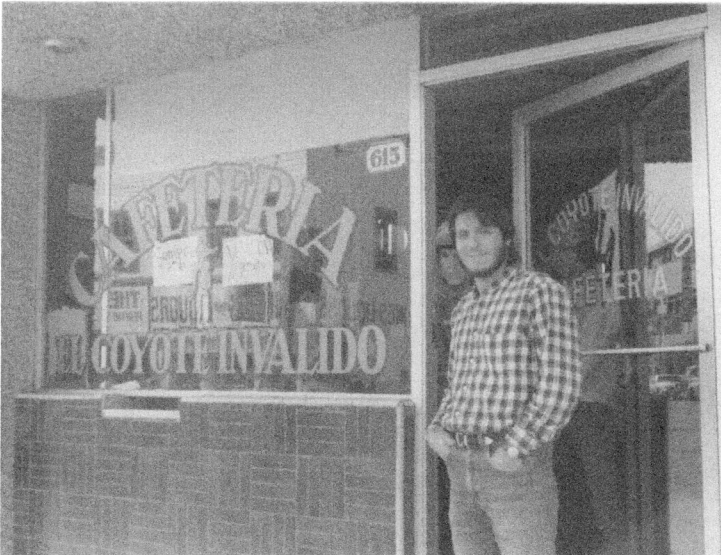

Me at lunch time out front of El Coyote Invalido, Cd Juarez, 1983

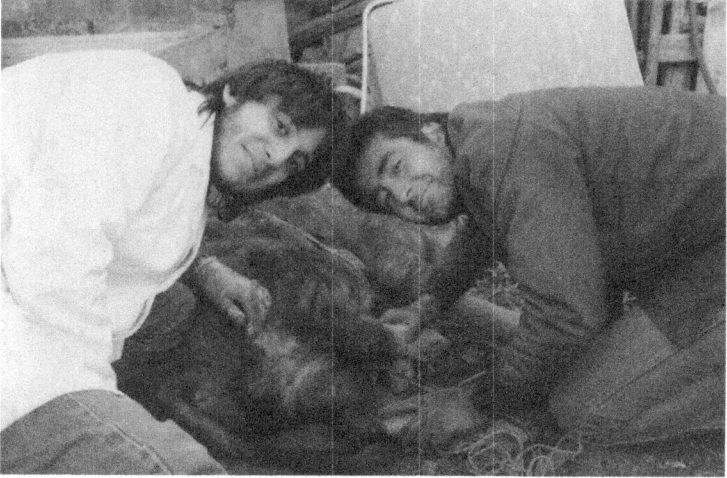

Alfonzo and I castrating his mother's pig, Cd. Jaurez 1983

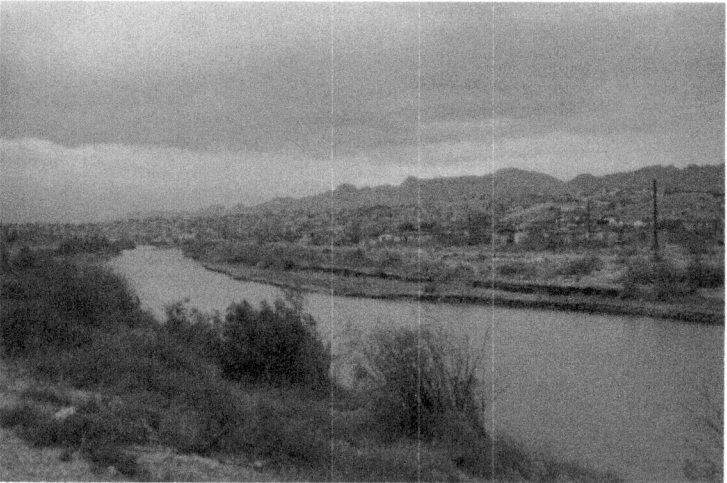

View of Rio Grande River and Cd. Jaurez in background. Picture taken from El Paso, Tx, 1983

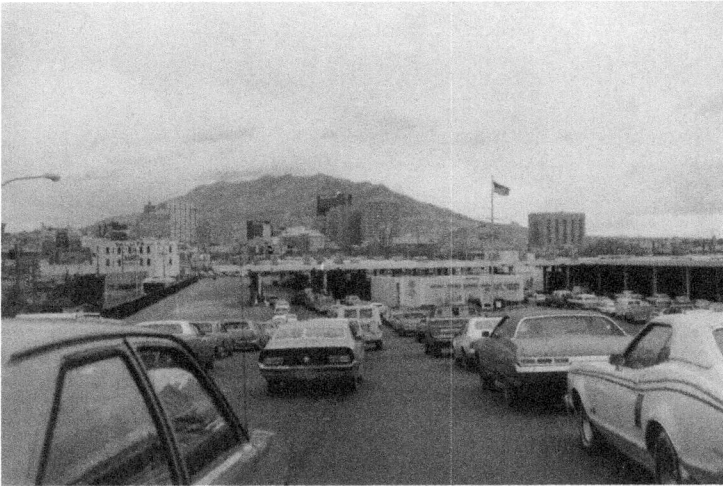

El Puente, the border crossing bridge for vehicles between El Paso, Tx
and Cd. Jaurez, Chihuahua, 1983.

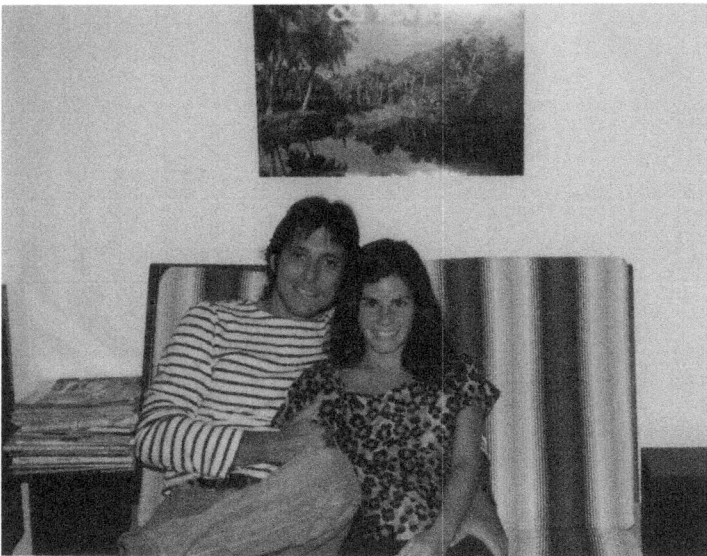

Mary Ellen and I at our Frigate Bay flat, 1984

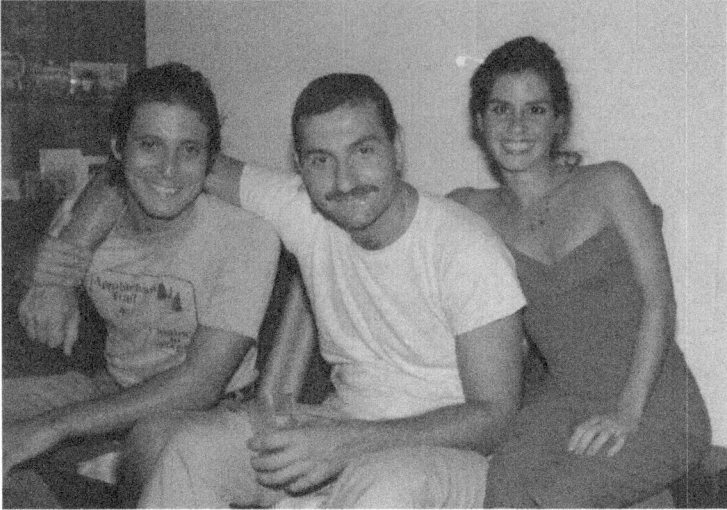

From left me, Lou Grasso and Mary Ellen in our flat overlooking Frigate
Bay, St, Kitts, 1984

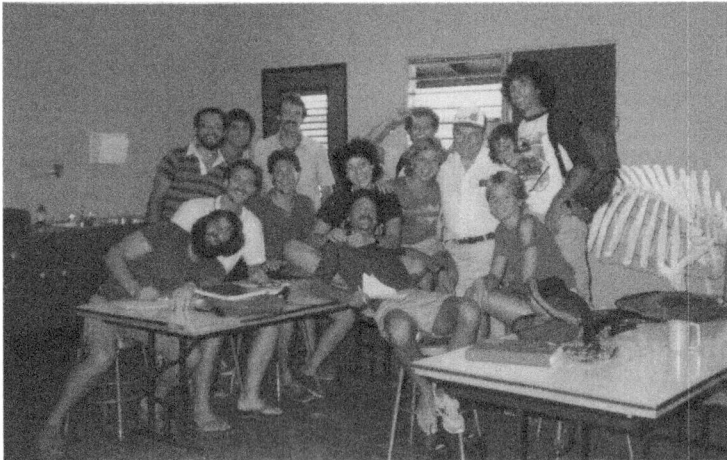

Classmates and Jesse Bone, DVM our anatomy professor inside Ross
University classroom spring 1984

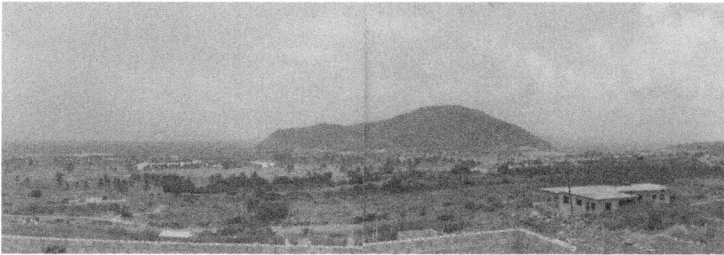

View from our apartment at Frigate Bay, St. Kitts. The Atlantic ocean viewed to the left of Timothy hill at center and the Caribbean sea is seen to the right of the hill, 1984

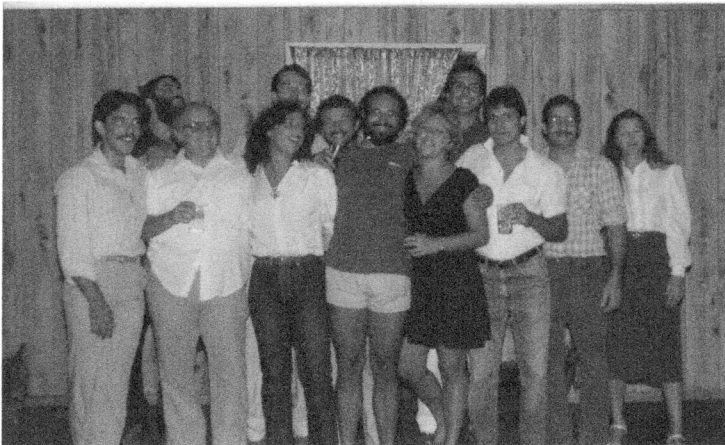

Classmates with Dr. Ronald Norman, professor of Parasitology, 1984

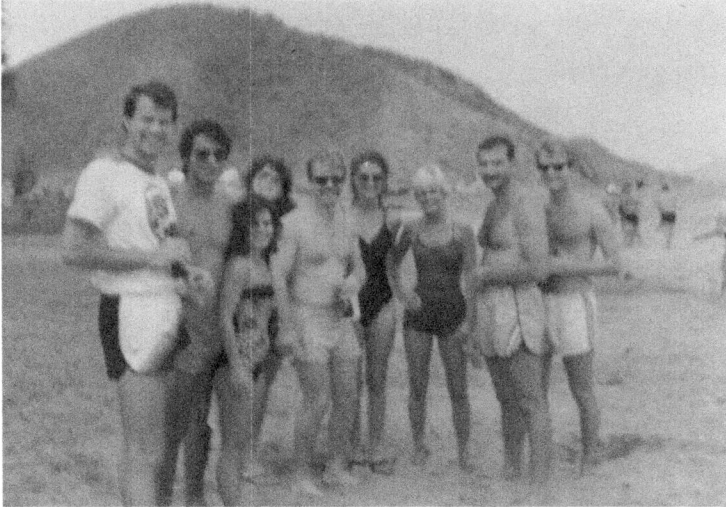

Classmates at beach party at "The Anchorage" on the Caribbean side.
MaryEllen and I are 3rd and 2nd from the left, 1984

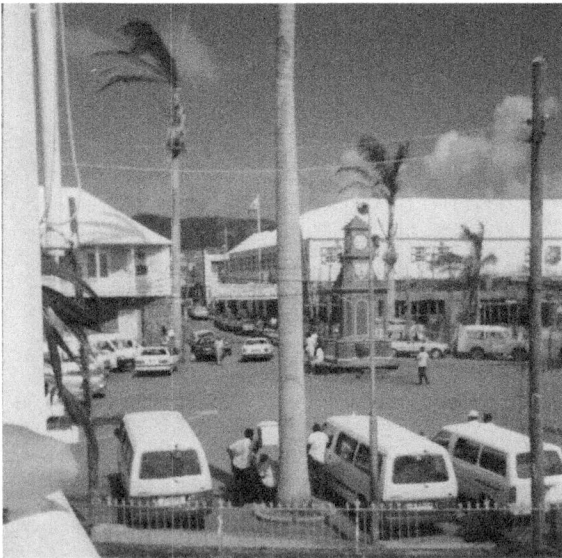

Downtown Bassettere, St. Kitts at the roundabout
called "The Circus," 1984

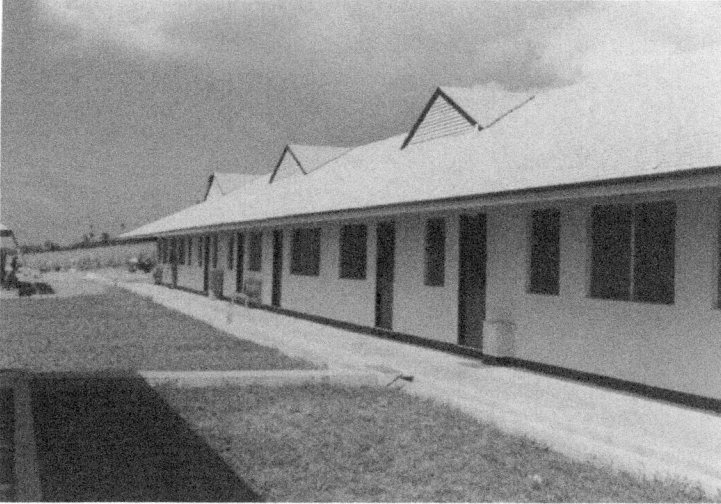

Typical outside view of some of the classrooms at Ross University,
School of Veterinary Medicine, St. Kitts, W.I. 1984

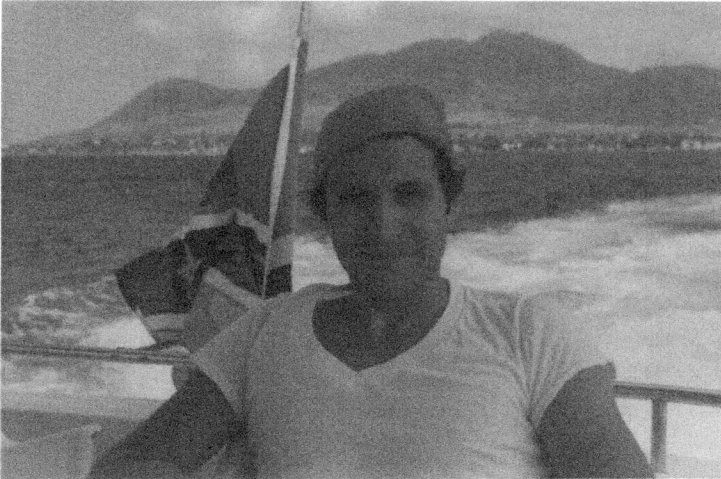

Boating along the southern coast of St. Kitts. At the rear, the two
star Kittian flag is flapping freely in the wind. The two stars
stand for St. Kitts and her sister island Nevis, 1984.

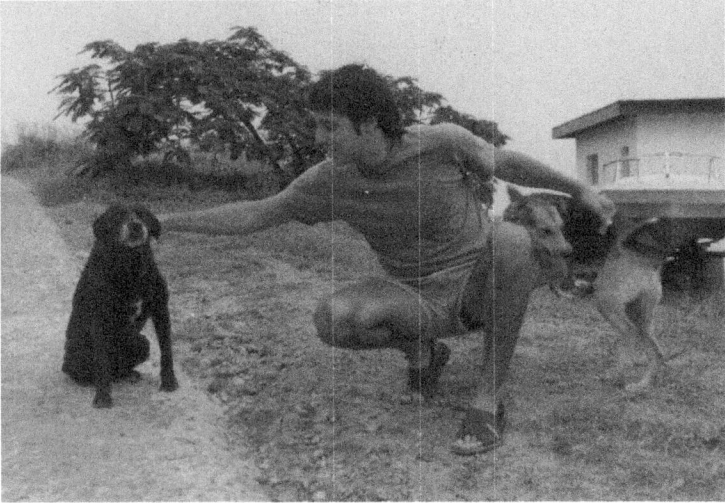

The Parlee's dogs "Patches" on my right and "Freddie"
on my left at home in St. Kitts, 1985.

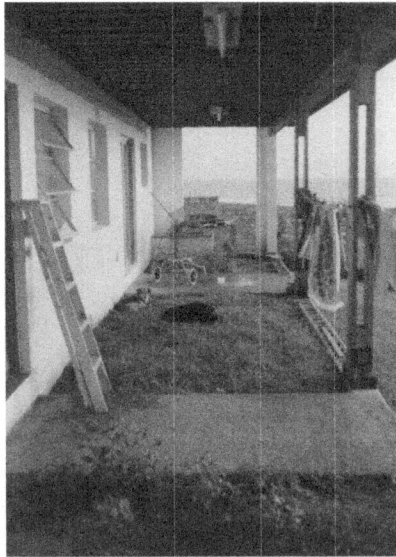

Outside our entrance to our Frigate Bay apartment. Note "Patches"
and "Freddie" keeping guard, 1985

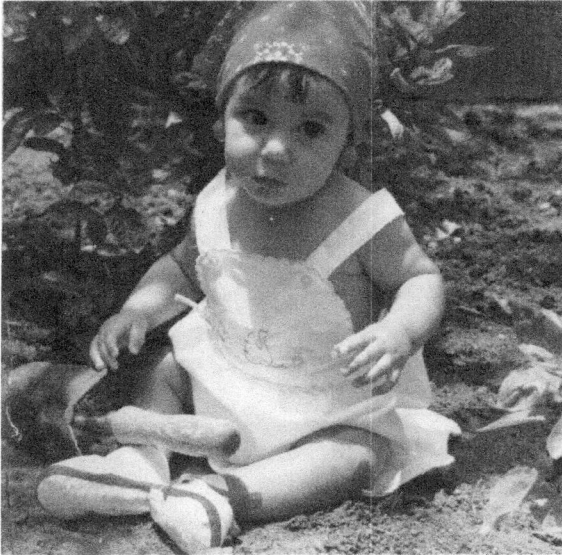

Jillian, our first born, picture that was an award winner in the Johnson
and Johnson Photo contest, 1986

The Board of Trustees, The President
and the members of the Class of June, 1987
of
Ross University School of Medicine
Ross University School of Veterinary Medicine
request the honor of your presence at the
Commencement Exercises
On Friday the Twelfth of June
At Six-thirty Post Meridien

Delegates Dining Room
United Nations Plaza
New York, New York

Commencement invitation for Ross University, School of Veterinary
Medicine graduation ceremony held at the Delegates Dining
room at the United Nations, NY, NY June 12 1987.

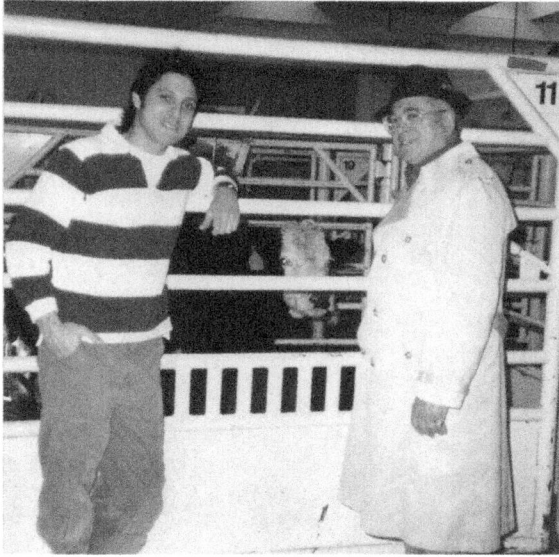

Dad and I in the Large Animal Hospital at Boren Veterinary Teaching
Hospital at Oklahoma State University, winter 1987.

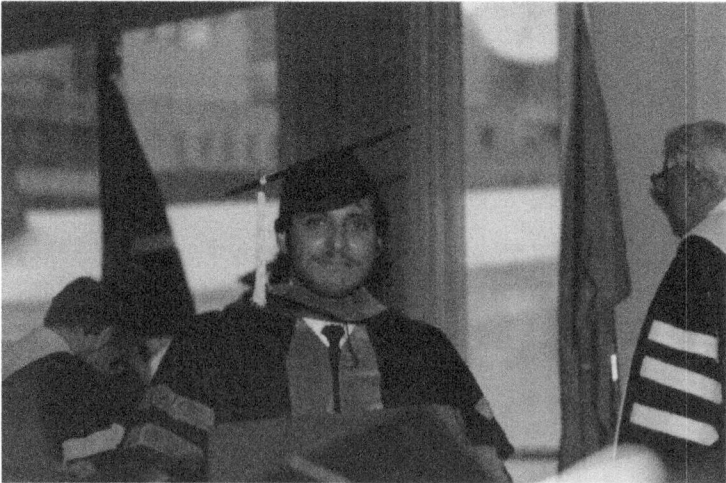

Me in graduation cap and gown, June 12, 1987

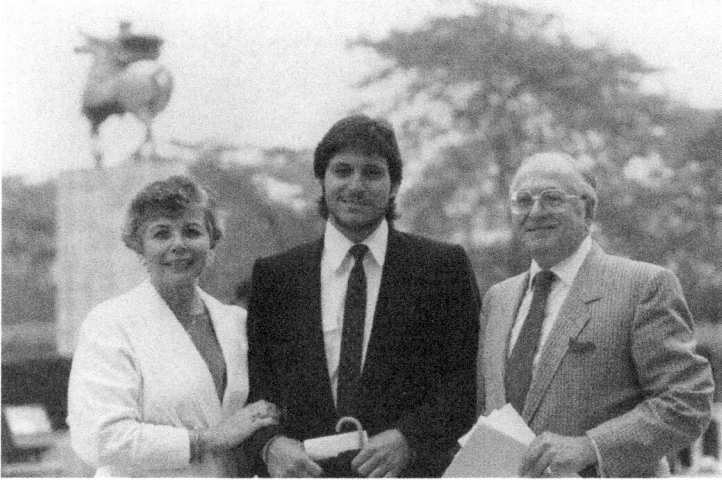

Mom, Dad and myself gathered outside the
United Nations Building, June 12, 1987.

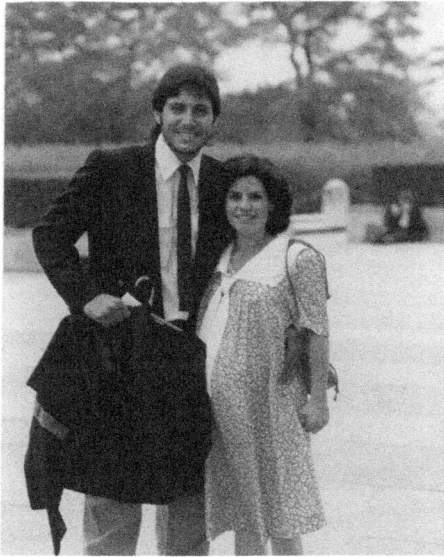

Mary Ellen 7 months pregnant with Abigail, and I outside the
United Nations Building, June 12, 1987

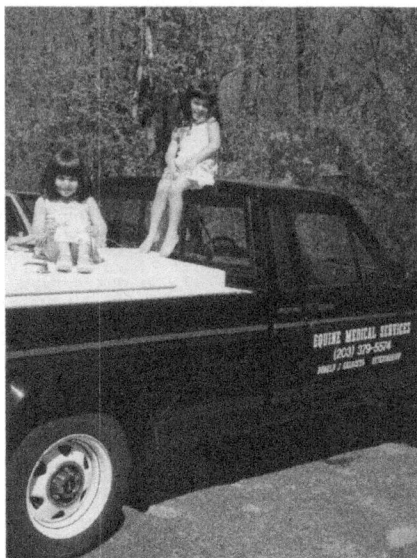

From left, Abigail and Jillian in 1990 playing on top of my mobile clinic during my equine practitioner days 1988 - 1995.

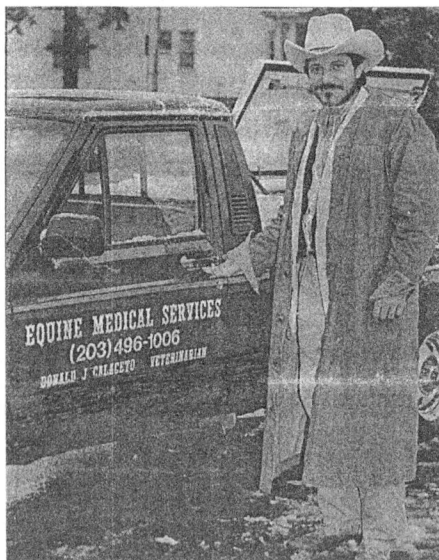

Photo that appeared in the Waterbury Republican, January 12, 1992 at the height of my equine practice.

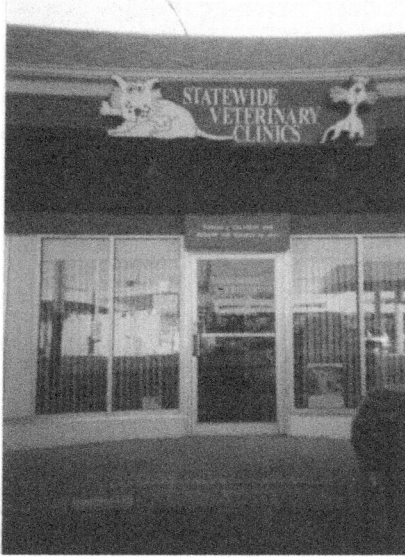

Statewide Veterinary Clinics, King St. Bristol, CT Dec. 1999 - Jan. 2008.

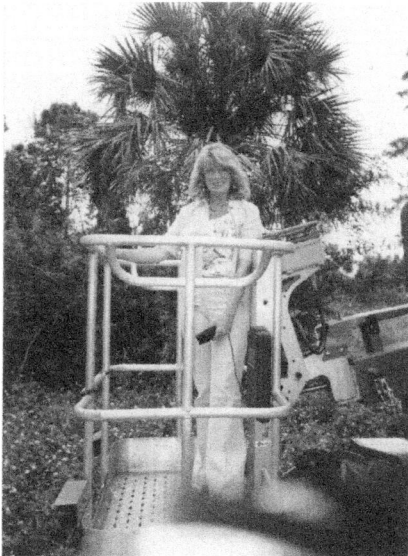

LuAnn after we purchased the land in 2003 for our new Florida home.
Picture was taken before raising the lift to enjoy our gulf view.

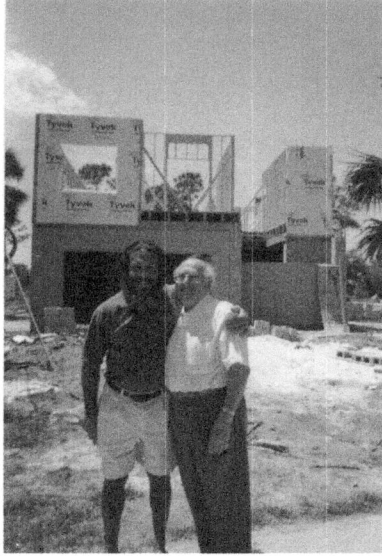

Dad and I outside the front of our Gulf house during construction, 2005.

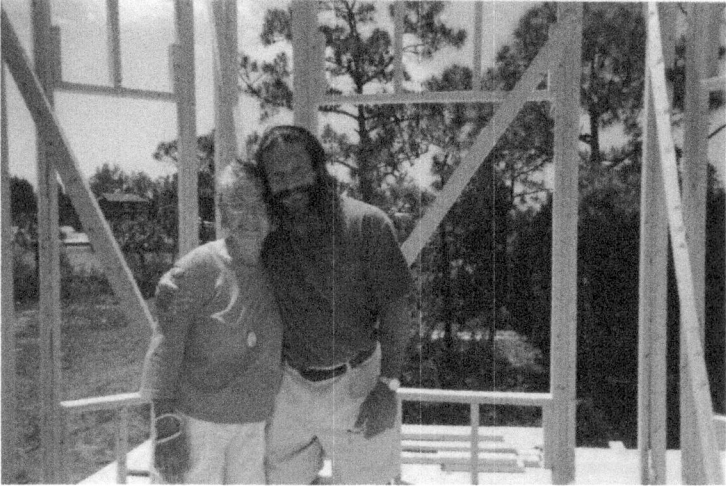

Mom and I in our future master suite during construction, 2005

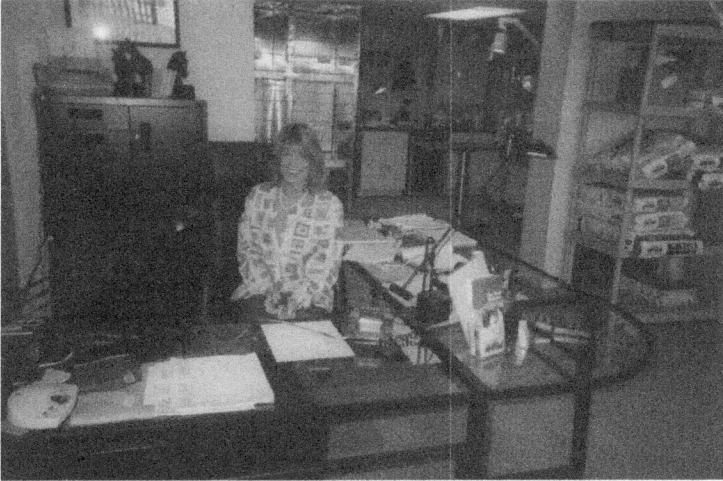

LuAnn, my wife working as my primary assistant at the
King St. office 2006-2007.

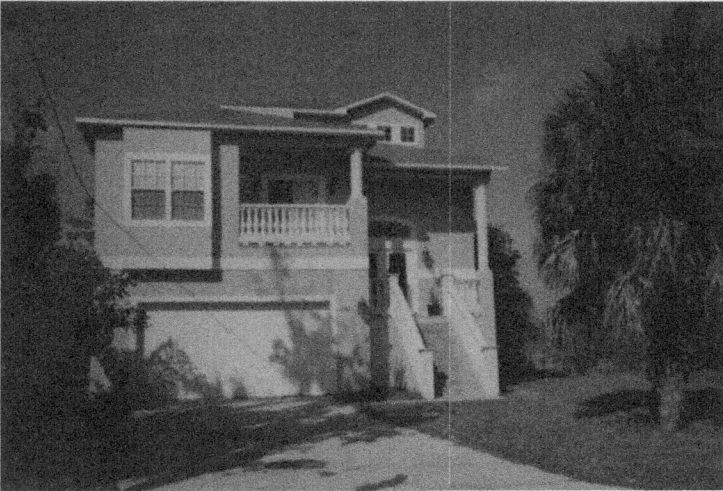

Front of Florida house after completion, 2007

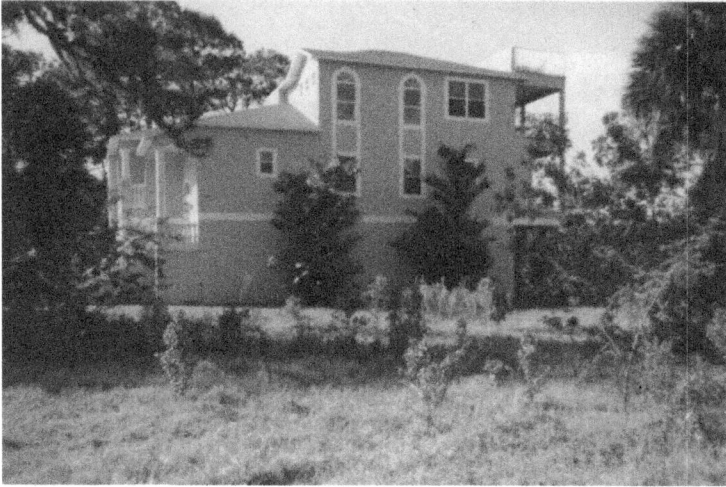

North side of Florida house after completion, 2007

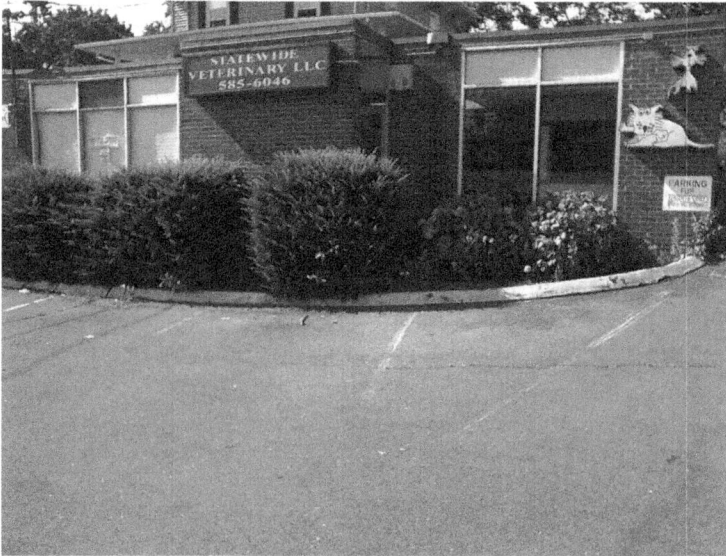

New Riverside Ave., Bristol office established on our return from Florida
June 2008 called Statewide Veterinary, LLC. Notice the word
Clinics was dropped from the title.

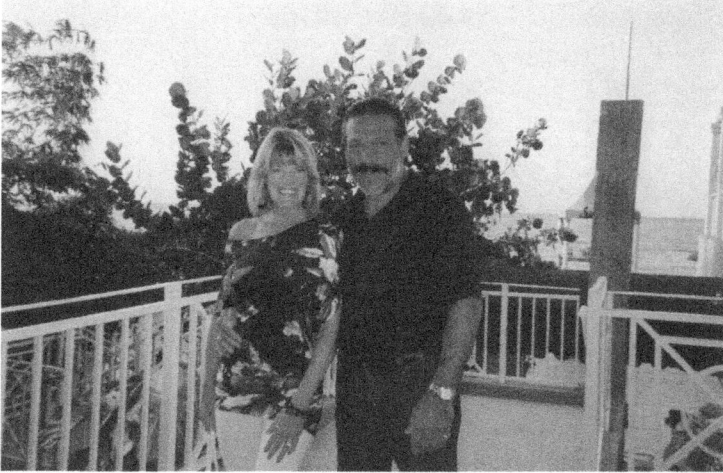

LuAnn and I at our Jamaican timeshare during the Labor Day holiday, 2011

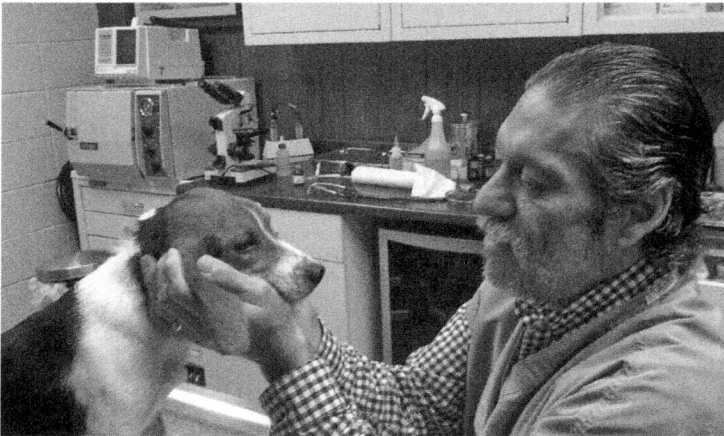

Pre-op exam/consultation with Maggie 5-20-14.

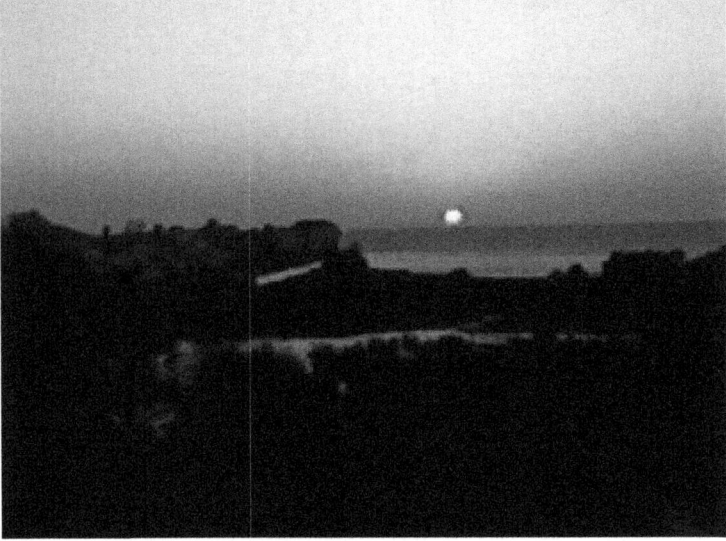

View of sunset from the upper deck of our Florida Gulf home.

PART II

FACTORS TO CONSIDER

L ast week a Borbeil Mastiff, who has not received regular veterinary care for financial reasons presented with advanced interdigital hemorrhagic mycotic dermatitis. This high priced pedigreed dog who has not been examined in years, is not receiving heartworm prevention and is only current on state required Rabies vaccination. Routine care including yearly examinations and inoculations have been disregarded.

Even purchasers of high priced pedigree dogs do not spend money for any regular veterinary care.

Ms. B and Mr. T were most anxious today under the circumstances to start treatment to alleviate his discomfort. But they were unprepared to pay for services which compromised the treatment plan and results. An anti-inflammatory injection, oral medication and an Elizabethan collar were recommended. The owner, who was short on funds had topical cream supplied for her own use that was applicable so I could save her some money on that portion of the treatment plan.

At check out, telecheck would not process their check. Mr. T came up with some cash to cover less than half of the invoice. I held on to the oral medication with a plan that they would show up in two days to pick it up. In fact it took them a week to raise $85.00 for the oral medication. By that time the long acting anti-inflammatory injection had worn off so the treatment plan was disrupted. Here is another example of inadequate funds to cover complete treatment so that animals are again left to suffer. This time because all the drugs in the treatment plan could not be started at the same time as intended.

When I saw them a week later, for a repeat injection that should have been two days sooner, to pick up the overdue oral medication I asked them a very important question.

How would you both vote if there is a question on the next ballot that asked if you would vote for national government regulated insurance for dogs and cats similar to Medicare for the aged and Medicaid for the underprivileged. They both said they would support that measure enthusiastically, in spite of the con-comitant increase in taxes that would have to be imposed to cover the cost of such a program. Ideally, we should mount a greater effort to find a government regulated national veterinary health plan that is adaptable to all income stratas. But it's better to walk away from the table with somethinglike Medicaid and Medicare to at least get started in this effort and at a later date make improvements. It's taken 47 years since the inception of Medicare for health care for all age groups and incomes to be a number one priority in the white house. We should try to add dog and cats to the "coat tails" of this movement as part of a Family health plan, but I suspect that the adoption of dog and cat governed programs may take at least as many years to orches-trate. Firstly, dogs and cats may have to be officially labeled as members of the family before they can be a part of the family health plan. The public in any event needs to voice their support for government intervention before a method can be devised. Legislatures will need to be informed of the inadequacies in care provided by many private low cost provider veterinary service operations as detailed in the this book, i.e. the use of chemical restraint without conventional anesthesia for low cost spays and neuters, absent exams that do not diagnose or treat common dis-eases that must be stopped and avoided, inferior diagnostic and treatment protocols due to financial constraints to mention a few so that these types of inferior services will not be advocated and reimbursed and therefore cease to operate.

Fortunately, my informal survey concludes that there is biparti-san agreement that we need government regulated national health care for people and their pets so it's possible with an orga-nized movement that public policy can be made for our com-panion animals too.

We should find a more affordable way for the government to finance Medicare and Medicaid before we can take on our house

pets. Second to the Military, health care is the next major cause
of our mounting national debt. Government insurance models
designed to pay for the promotion of human health i.e. by providing coverage for routine tests and treatments for common
diseases will have to adopted for veterinary care because routine
diagnostic tests and treatment procedures done early in the
pathogenesis of disease ultimately will save the taxpayer money
while improving the quality of animal care.

For example heartworm and gastrointestinal endoparasite
screenings as needed, and juvenile spays and neuters done on a
recommended schedule can save lives and large sums of money
in treatment care. If a female is not spayed when she is young she
will often develop Pymoetra, a costly disease to treat, or worse
metastatic mammary adenocarcinoma, a form of cancer that will
end her life. Parasites if not stopped early in their development
cause severe debilitation and much more costly treatment
regimes to be put in place.

More costly orthopedic, ophthalmic and dental procedures and
benign tumor removals that affect the quality of an otherwise
healthy animal will have to be included in the plan to stop
unnecessary long term medical costs and stop animal suffering.
If entropion, inward folding of the eyelids, can be corrected
when they are puppies and kittens, secondary corneal diseases,
can be avoided that require lengthy and more costly long term
treatment protocols. If the practitioner knows that he will be
reimbursed for the diagnostic and treatment procedures that
need to be performed, and the owners know that they are not
expected to reach deeply into their pocket at the time of services
or that government relief is on its way to assist in payment, there
will no longer be owner neglect or interference with the practice
of veterinary medicine as it should be. I had hoped after the
advent of private pet insurance that there would have been a
marked increase in the delivery of higher quality veterinary services but I have been sadly disappointed.

Currently private pet insurance is not reimbursing sufficiently for the procedures required, because their first priority is to make a profit. Limited reimbursement by private insurance providers, is not solving the problem because many owners are not getting adequate financial reimbursement to risk their financial security paying upfront for all services needed. As a result, most of my clients do not even choose to keep private veterinary insurance because they've experienced inadequate reimbursement, they can not afford the premiums, and because no upfront money is guaranteed by private insurance.

Some time ago, a 11 y A/M Rottweiller presented with inappetance, rhinitis, and a firm swelling at the area of the left frontal sinus (forehead). After unsuccessful conservative treatment with antibacterial and NSAIDS, I convinced the owner to try surgical removal. She had private veterinary insurance, but since they do not provide upfront money to cover procedure costs, she couldn't afford the pre-op blood work or the biopsy I recommended. Those test would have added at least another 275.00 to her bill. In reality that is a small price to pay for valuable information.

Without a biopsy, I did not have the opportunity to have the pathologist determine if the mass that was attached to the left side of the frontal bone was benign, malignant, and/or infectious in character. After two surgeries which included penetration of the left frontal sinus to remove the bone attached mass, the dog improved but later developed a similar mass over the right side of the frontal bone. If cytology from the biopsy revealed fungus, possibly a long course of antifungal therapy may have successfully treated the problem. If the mass was determined to be malignant by the pathologist with a grave prognosis, I would have put the dog to sleep to end his suffering. To better determine a definitive course of action we need sufficient payment to perform the procedures we require. An arrangement between the government and the veterinarian for reimbursement or tax relief for the owner would have made it possible to receive payment for pre-op. lab work and a biopsy as recommended and a diagnosis/prognosis rendered that would have caused less suffering for the animal and owner.

When the second mass developed, the owner and I agreed to euthanasia. From the beginning to the end she spent 1770.00 on treatment. After multiple submissions of documents to her private insurance company she only received 650.00 as reimbursement for her veterinary costs.

It is typical for private insurance companies to short change their policy holders like this. This causes owners to stop policies and word to spread about deficient reimbursement so that potential applicants do not seek private pet insurance. With or without private insurance coverage, often we do not get enough money upfront when the patient is admitted to practice quality medicine and surgery as we should.

What's the alternative? Just euthanize these cases to stop suffering because there isn't enough money to practice higher quality medicine to prevent these sorts of results?

Not acceptable.

Government assistance has to happen

Yesterday Mrs. C called about her 14y Lhasa who was very uncomfortable with an interdigial cyst-like lesion on his left hind leg. Before admitting the dog for surgery, I pointed out to Mr. C. that the dog still desperately needed a long overdue dental that most likely will include some extractions. I told him since I needed to anesthetize the dog today that today would be an excellent time to include this overdue procedure. He chose to ignore the problem because he did not have enough funds to cover both procedures. After the foot surgery while still under anesthesia, I took the opportunity to examine his mouth and immediately found an upper left molar that was in urgent need of extraction. Later when he picked up the dog, I mentioned this finding and again he chose to ignore the problem.

This dog is obviously uncomfortable and yet nothing is done because the owner is not able to pay upfront or otherwise. It's not that I was going to require him to pay for costly crown fillings or root canal. I just wanted to increase the estimate by two or three hundred dollars so I could take the opportunity to extract any teeth causing pain and remove tartar on the rest of the remaining teeth. Many animals are suffering from painful dental disease, because many owners can not even afford to pay for the extraction of teeth causing this pain.

People are not prepared to pay for their own health care or their pet's healthcare. They depend on the state or federal insurance programs in many cases to assist them when the private insurance carrier finds excuses not to reimburse the hospitals, doctors, laboratories and pharmacies.

When I finished the first edition of this book, I faced a new kind of challenge. I was diagnosed with Myasthenia gravis after emergency admission to the hospital for respiratory insufficiency. I was kept on a respirator for five days until I could breathe on my own. A disabling neuromuscular autoimmune disease caused by antibodies produced against Acetylcholine receptors which results in blocking neuromuscular impulses.

This disease, uncontrolled by medication causes widespread muscular distress. Insufficient innervation to my tongue for six. months caused me to loose speech and the ability to swallow many foods resulting in 50# weight loss and the inability to speak with my clientele. My personal experience with human medical care since my admission to the hospital has alerted me to the same flaws in the delivery of medical insurance coverage to people as well.. For instance, to not pay out, my insurance company claimed that I had a pre-diagnosed condition before the treatments began.

Even though I was paying a private insurance carrier premiums monthly, they chose not to pay out to anyone that helped save my life. Fortunately, I was treated and discharged before the hospital and I knew that the insurance company would deny coverage, otherwise I may have not received care and passed away like a dog or cat.

An attorney who thought my case was hopeless referred me to the Health Care Advocate who was unsuccessful in my defense.

Greed and profits instead of saving lives are the priority of both the human and companion animal insurance companies. Veterinary insurance companies employ the same tactics to find any reason they can to deny claims insisting that insured dogs and cats have pre diagnosed conditions.
They will request records from my office to find any questionable notes to build a case to deny coverage.
Ultimately, the patient must receive treatment and the doctors, hospitals and staff must be paid. Currently, the government usually ends up paying a lower rate of compensation for the treatment of uninsured human hospital patients. Why not do the same for our pets?

Because they do not, veterinarians are expected to forgo routine treatment protocol and conveniently euthanize pets whenever funds are not available to save them. Furthermore to do so, some veterinarians can be caught speculating fictiously after a cursory exam that their medical conditions are terminal to ease the pet owner's conscience. This should be a very disturbing fact to any learned pet owner.

Government agencies to guarantee funds or to put institutions in place to provide treatments can stop this falsehood.

Given the chance, some other necessary treatments which should be conveniently done while a patient is under anesthesia such as dental extractions, tumor removals, etc. are omitted.

Sometimes even pre-op blood work is denied at a potentially great risk to the patient, to limit costs to the owner just to make any surgery affordable.

A 8y spayed Golden Retriever came in for eyelid surgery yesterday. She was scheduled for later this week but the condition got unmanageable for the owner because the masses to be excised were becoming much larger and irritated. The surgery was originally postponed because the owner needed to raise the 500.00 to cover the General anesthetic the procedure and necessary medication. Pre-op bloodwork and biopsy costs were denied and omitted because they were not affordable. The eyelid was so swollen that I administered a Triamcinalone anti-inflammatory injection pre-op so that the masses would reduce to a more reasonable operable size by the time I commenced surgery. They reduced considerably after about 1 hour and we performed an uneventful procedure. At the end of the day the dog appeared weaker and less alert than usual but the vital signs were relatively normal. The dog was released at approximately 5:30. She walked out to the car without a lively step, but I attributed her lack of enthusiasm to her discomfort, high level of emotion and recent surgery. Later at approximately 8:15 P.M. , the owner called that she had died after she had defacated large black stools. It is quite possible that if I could have performed pre-op blood work and a stool examination that this unfortunate event could have been avoided.

Without lab confirmation I can only speculate that the dog had pancreatic and/or liver disease and reacted to the Tiamcinalone injection which eventually caused the dog to go into shock. I have known this dog for five years and after taking many histories the owner never told me about loose or black stools and any vomiting.

Now that I was aware of these stools I asked him if if he had been observing these black stools episodically and or recently and he said he didn't know because the dog defacates in the back yard and he does not check the character of the stools. Incidentally, the same owner had a another dog that died approximately nine years ago from Pancreatic Disease. In fact he did not tell me about the table scraps she received until she passed. I went on to ask him if this dog was in the habit of receiving table scraps against my advice like the last dog. He said that he and his wife were not giving table food but he wasn't sure about his 4 yr old son. Months later his wife told me that after I asked them to conduct a search that they found many black stools in the backyard. I obviously can't control how a pet is cared for in the home, but if insurance was in force that would pay for routine pre-op blood and other required tests, i.e. radiographs, fecal exams, etc. this death could have been avoided. Another way this outcome might be avoided is to receive sincere and complete histories from owners. Some owners, in an effort to keep costs down, are reluctant to advise me of valuable histories that would cause me to insist on pre-op diagnostics workups.

Many conditions such as pancreatic and heart attacks can be avoided if an owner would convey a true history of their pets. Ms. R brought her daughters dog to my office for the first time two weeks ago.

This six year old Rottweiler cross was lazy with allopecia at the tail head and bridge of the nose. A Heartworm neg. test and very low T4 was found, in addition to two causes of lameness. Thyrosyn and a NSAID were dispensed and one week later the owner called to congratulate me on the Hypothyroidism and lameness diagnosis and told me the dog was doing much better on the medical treatment. One week after that I got a telephone call to learned that the dog suddenly died. After I kindly cross examined her daughter about the dog I learned that she was exercising him more since he was feeling better and that he would tire easily. In fact he would walk just two short blocks and have to rest. Her daughter thought that this was because he was out of shape and that after continued work outs he would get in better physical shape.

Wrong.

Eventhough his heart valves and rhythm were normal on auscultation, I suspect his myocardium was not.

A valuable history may have been taken on this dog if the daughter came in with the dog. In that case, if money was not an obstacle or government insurance available, chest radiographs would have been taken that may have shown an enlarged heart, or an ultrasound may have revealed myocardial disease.

Medication for the heart as well as the other medications would have been dispensed with instruction for limited exercise, and her dog would be alive and medically managed successfully. I suspect if Mrs. R knew of the dog's exercise intolerance that she did not volunteer the information to save money on the yearly check up costs.

As it should be, it is typical before we as humans have surgery or receive certain treatments that certain tests are run. Why and how is this possible? Because they should be and because the government and private insurance companies are usually covering the costs for these tests. If we didn't have government or private insurance companies promising payment directly to our care providers, most of us wouldn't receive these pre treatment tests either, and procedures performed on us and drugs prescribed would be as risky as it is for our pets .

Currently, unlike human private medical insurance coverage, private animal insurance plans do not work because all animal insurance plans presently require the owner to pay upfront for all services rendered.

Furthermore, animal insurance companies want to dictate what procedures need to be done and limit reimbursement because their main objective is to turn as much profit as possible from every animal receiving treatment.

They know the veterinarian has been paid. They are only confronted by the ignorant and confused pet owner for reimbursement, who isn't trained and experienced in veterinary care to present an argument to justify the cost of procedures that needed to be done on the patient's behalf.

Since the government has more altruistic motives than the profit driven private sector, they are needed to assist in the design of reimbursement models based on typical treatment protocols and regulate private insurance practices and/or administer their own insurance programs so that so that dogs and cats are treated humanely and practitioners are reimbursed sufficiently. How are veterinarian able to practice with the skills and experience they have acquired when the animal's care depends on payment which is not immediately available or guaranteed. Yesterday I was presented with another frustrating situation.

Mr. B presented a dog who I was treating for Lymes disease that had not eaten in four days.

This 8 year old spayed Black lab was also continually vomiting even though water and food were not taken in the last 36 hours. The owner said he had very limited funds to allocate for veterinary care.

The dog was moribund, and approximately 10 percent dehydrated. Blood was immediately drawn and and I.V. drip started and antibiotic and anitemetic injectibles administered.   The budget was 350.00. After two liters of fluids and medication by injection she was more alert, but still in desperate need of extended hospitalization with intensive care. Since the owner could not afford that, she was discharged with instructions for nothing per os and rest until the lab work results could be obtained tomorrow a.m..

Lab results revealed severe pancreatitis, Diabetes, renal compromise and infection indicated by a marked increase in the absolute white count and bands. I immediately called the owner to advise him of the dog's condition. He was upset mostly because he had to listen to his dog moan from discomfort through the night because he couldn't afford to hospitalize the dog with me.

Because he couldn't afford hospital care for his dog both he and the dog suffered. The dog suffered from his medical condition and the owner suffered emotionally because he had to watch his dog suffer.

Hospitals for the invalid, provide treatment for the animals and a place where pets can be kept so that family members are spared the agony of watching their diseased pets. Later the same day he called me in distress to inform me the dog had died, and that he wanted to bring her to my office for disposal. I immediately met and expressed my sympathy and heart felt understanding. Then I had to charge him 90.00 for storage and mass cremation. The total bill 440.00 for the entire scenario. So. Here we have an owner stifled by 440.00 spent in a 24 hour period that was insufficient to properly take care of this dog.

This dog should have received extended hospitalization, follow up blood work taken, and I.V. fluids, insulin, and further I.V. antibiotic injections and whatever else was needed given. But if the intensive care that was required was administered for an extended hospital stay his bill would have been beyond his reach and we would not have been reimbursed to pay our expenses. On the other hand, some clients can afford a three day hospitalization stay to find a diagnosis and to stabilize the patient before discharge. They can even afford long term medication for six weeks to treat Heptitis as is the Case with Mr. D. but they can't handle the home nursing care the pet requires to recover.

Mr. D. presented his 10y s/f lab cross 2 ½ weeks ago. She stayed with me for three days and was discharged with medication to treat hepatitis and a fair prognosis. Almost every other day the owner would call to complain about how difficult it was to take

care of his dog in this condition. I continually reminded him
that there would be a very slow recovery and that he needed to
be patient. The dog was weak, eating a little, drinking sufficient
water, and not vomiting. I was convinced she was receiving all
his medication as prescribed. A few days ago on Friday at 6
A.M., he left me a message implying that he wanted to euthanize
the dog. We offered to hospitalize the dog for further evaluation
and care so that they would not have to care for her for the
weekend.   But the owner decided to take the dog to his
boyfriend's veterinarian about 1 hour away for another opinion.
By now I think you might know what treatment answer this
owner was looking for.

Anyway, we faxed the lab work which indicated minor elevations
in liver enzymes and that was the end of that. Because affordable extended hospital care is not available this dog was euthanized by another veterinarian who chose to accommodate their
request. All this dog needed was a stable environment away from
his owner and money to cover the costs for at least two weeks
conservative hospital care to recover.

Owners usually can not emotionally handle the task of extended
home nursing care for their weakened pets. Again the veterinarian is expected to put an animal to sleep to end the owner's
misery. Not the pet's misery. Either owners can not handle the
emotional aspects of extended home nursing, or they can not
afford the cost of extended veterinary care, even when the prognosis is good. The following owner could not handle either
aspect of the equation even when the prognosis is good.

Recently, 12.5y spayed female Yellow LabX presented. The
owner stated that she was not herself since she ingested rancid
food approximately six months ago. The physical exam findings
revealed an elevated body temperature, hind end lameness, and
overall weakness.. I recommended blood work and radiographs
to aid toward reaching a diagnostic and treatment plan.. She was
not willing to spend money for radiographs, but was willing to

pay for lab work.. But she was very interested in euthanasia.. I was not.

Nothing unusual about that.

I took the case because I wanted the dog to have a chance, .and because I made the owner aware of the limitations she imposed on me to practice the highest quality veterinary medicine.

Because there is no government insurance to help the financially disabled or uncooperative pet owner to pay for the costs for all the diagnostic testing, this situation is far too common causing inaccurate assessments and substandard treatment results. The white blood cell count and a specific liver enzymes were found elevated. I suggested radiographs again because a nonspecific liver enzyme (alkaline phosphate) was so elevated that there may have been a tumor. She was not interested, except to pay for any medication that might help.

Antibiotics and liver supplement were prescribed and instructions to return for follow up blood work in 30 days. I told her that with hepatitis she would be weak and that there would be at least a 3-6 months period of convalescence.

When she returned with the dog she was encouraged with the treatment results The dog was more alert and there was no more putrid smelling flatulence.. The second round of blood work included additional cost for total and direct (conjugated) bilirubin to determine cause(s) of the hepatitis. The owner complained about the additional expense and I absorbed the additional cost. This lab work revealed some valuable information.

The results revealed a significant drop in the live enzymes, a significant increase in white blood cell count, a considerable drop in red blood cell count and 100% indirect (unconjugated bilirubin). The results were indicative of hemolytic disease, defined as a disease that destroys red blood cells. The cause of the hemolytic disease still needed to be determined before the best treatment could be put in place.

I then determined that I needed to do testing for autoimmune hemolytic disease, but again the owner continued that she did not want to pay for any more lab work.. She begrudgingly picked up the Doxycycline I prescribed to treat infection hemolytic disease. I could not justify dispensing medication to treat for autoimmune hemolytic disease without lab confirmation.

No radiographs and no testing for autoimmune disease had probably compromised the care of this dog but by this time it was obvious that the treatment on board was the best care that this owner was willing to pay for. Fortunately the dog continued improved on the treatment I prescribed.

The whole time the owner was repeatedly complaining about having to help the dog rise because of his lame back end. I kept telling her that I would not dispense medication for the purpose because it could compromise her liver function.

Finally about a month after the second round of blood work I gave in because I felt that they might give up on this dog. I prescribed a conservative dose schedule with a non steroidal anti-inflammatory drug (NSAID), with strict instructions to call with a progress report in seven days, and to discontinue it immediately and call if the medication caused any set back.

Her husband called me three weeks later and told me she had a terrible setback and that he wanted to euthanize her. Meanwhile, he was still giving the NSAID. I told him it was possibly due to the use of the NSAID I advised against. I asked him why he didn't stop the NSAID and why he waited so long to call me. Maybe he was thinking the "she was just a dog". I told him to stop the NSAID and to call in five days with a progress report. I never heard from them again.

They didn't want to pay for the treatment this dog required and they did not want to be inconvenienced by his weakness. The cause of the drama with the following case was only financial.

Mrs. H approximately 8 weeks ago brought her 9 mos. Altered male chocolate lab. Radiographs revealed that he had simple metacarpal fractures across his right front paw after his foot was crushed by a car. Her dog was anesthetized, radiographs taken and the lower leg placed in a cast to include the toes.

She had to borrow money from her mother because she didn't have enough upfront money to pay for the procedure. Ten days ago she called me and wanted to know what it would cost for her return visit for cast removal. I told her that I would need to first take radiographs of the foot to check for sufficient union of the bones involved. If healing was sufficient, I then would administer chemical restraint to the dog before removing the cast with a power saw. If the cast was to be removed, I gave her a total estimate of approximately 250.00.

The appointment for the evaluation would have been this morning, but her husband called yesterday to inform me that he was canceling the appointment because he had already removed the cast. Why?

Obviously to save money.

But guess what?

There may have been insufficient callus formation to support the healed fracture, and if so the the site will refracture. Removing the cast after 6 and 1/2 weeks may have been too soon for an adequate callus formation to stabilize the fractures. Radiographic evaluation of the site is mandatory before cast removal.

If insurance was in force to cover the costs of re-evaluation and treatments i.e. sedation, radiographs and cast removal, he would not have taken control of this situation and put his dogs health in jeopardy. The way to ensure that medical and surgical protocols are followed and prevent most unnecessary animal suffering is to make sure that government regulated insurance can pay for the services. Federal Taxes will have to be collected and allocated when an owner is financially disadvantaged or tax deductions allowed to assist the struggling middle class. Then if need be to enforce responsible conduct, owners can be charged with animal cruelty if our instructions are not followed. Currently insufficient money to pay for services is a common excuse for animal neglect and suffering. To have the most affect, we need to get the federal government involved in the health care of our dogs and cats to establish nationwide criteria for animal health care and the prevention of pet cruelty.

Eventhough, guaranteed financial support is the goal for all veterinary services, we can start in this effort by getting federal government assistance by allowing a sizeable schedule A tax deduction for the middle class majority for spaying and neutering our dogs and cats. If a sizeable enough tax credit is put in place that could cover cat and dog spays and neuters done under conventional anesthetic, then owners can seek out venues that perform safe painless procedures. A dog and cat can't speak to tell his owner how painful a poor quality surgical procedure was because of insufficient anesthetic depth, because cheaper less labor intensive Disassociative Anesthetic was used instead of conventional general gas anesthetic.

If owners are guaranteed reimbursement for the cost of a quality procedure than a quality procedure is what they will seek. Quality instead of cost will become the first priority.

Furthermore, once a large enough tax credit is in place to cover the cost of a safer and humane spay and neuter the way it should be done, it will be easier to get public cooperation to shut down low cost providers that spay and neuter using disassociative anesthesia.

We need to expand our interpretation of animal cruelty to include laws against unacceptable veterinary care.

To ensure that appropriate veterinary care is given for spays and neuters, specific animal protection laws for safe and humane spays and neuters have to be established and enforcement maintained before government regulated tax credits and insurance practices can effectively contribute towards correcting this situation.

Enforcement will have to include unannounced government inspections of low cost spay and neuter facilities to shut down those clinics that do not perform services at federal standards, to disqualify them as venues for owner tax credits and/or recipients of government funding.

Furthermore, tax credits for spays and neuters will have to be designed to ensure that the funding is per procedure to stop owners from trying to bargain with veterinarians for multiple pet discounts. Multiple pet discounting lends itself to incomplete and substandard services.

Since the labor and products cost the same, it is impossible to provide equivalent services for multiple animals at reduced prices. An establishment that offers multiple pet discounts does so at a loss to personal income or at a loss to the quality in the delivery of animal medial care. Which do you think is going to happen?

Unfortunately, without government laws and financial assistance, the private sector will continue to make the wrong choices because making a profit or saving money is usually the first priority. The government will need to distribute funds for the public directly to practitioners such as the case with Medicaid, to ensure that the money will be used as intended. We can not always trust people to spend money as instructed.

For example food stamps should not be used to purchase alcoholic beverages and welfare checks should not be used to encourage a gambling or drug addiction. People have proven time and time again to abuse financial assistance programs. Therefore if the government is to help with payment of veterinary care it may have to issue identification cards so these funds can only be used for that purpose. Furthermore veterinarians will have to be held accountable for their services in order to be paid. The federal government should set the course with animal cruelty laws and assistance so that the quality of animal health care will be equivalent nationwide.

Federal offices similar to those designed to operate the Medicare and Medicaid programs need to be run to improve animal medical and surgical services. May I suggest that we call it Veticare and Veticaid. To help the aged and increasing financially disadvantaged pet owner population to properly care for their family pets. We all sympathize with the needs of the aged, disabled and poor. But what do we think about the working middle class of this country that is financially incapable of paying for quality veterinary medical and surgical care? Should we put liens on their homes or force them to sell their homes to pay their debts?

Human and pet illness costs do not justify putting hard working middle class people in the street.

The costs of medical and surgical care has climbed so high as to cause liens and losses of family estates. Does that imply that the inability to pay medical costs have the capacity to eventually cause the disownership of property by the taxpayer in this country if we do not define boundaries to creditor collection practices?

Yes, I am afraid it does.

Has veterinary care not been able to recognize government financial support thus far because human medical government assistance has not been managed successfully? Possibly.

By allowing the creation of huge medical debt and subsequent loss of property titles and property tax revenue from the middle class of this country who can not afford medical care, the government has in affect partnered with the medical providers/industry and banks to shrink our middle class economy. The middle class typically looses their titles after defaulting on second and third mortgages and credit cards used to try to pay off these unaffordable medical debts.

The remaining upper and upper middle class managing to hold on to their titles of ownership are paying increasing property and income taxes to help the government make payments on loans they have taken out to cover the lost tax revenue from the bourgeois whom have lost their homes and jobs.

Most of the homeowners that manage to keep up with the interest payments on these loans are not able to sufficiently reduce their principal balances in their working lifetime so that when they die their houses are sold to pay off these unpaid debts. In many cases these homes end up with large liens that cause these properties to be foreclosed upon and the delinquent taxes are not paid increasing government liabilities.

Banks do not accept responsibility and pay back taxes on foreclosed properties.

Only if there is a new homeowner who needs excellent credit to qualify for a mortgage will the government receive the unpaid taxes. The U.S. banks whom borrow, lend and invest money on margin have obvious financial instability. As proof, just remember the consequences of the Over the Counter Derivatives and Sub Prime Lending that occurred before and after the millennium respectively. The government has had to put the taxpayer's financial health at risk causing them to loose their credit in too many cases, because they have had to borrow money and increase taxes to make payments to bail out the banks on numerous occasions.

Obama claims that our national debt has tripled during the Obama administration largely to bail out overextended U.S. banks, in hopes of stimulating the economy. But new mortgages or any other credit will not get approved for our increasing population of middle class non credit worthy applicants. I suggest a "Forgiveness Act" for the Middle Class so that many more applicants can qualify for the "stimulus money" that was given to the banks, because new loans to the middle class will generate more tax revenue to help pay down government debt.

Meanwhile the world banks, including China that have been continuously lending our government funds to pay for our mounting medical debt, may eventually own most of this country if we can't find a workable solution to health care costs and unchecked self centered banking practices. The federal government may not have the financial strength to take on veterinary care until they can pay down their debt, generate more tax revenue to pay expenses and better manage their books on human healthcare costs.

We and the animals we love are the victims of the mounting interest payments the U.S. government is making on foreign country loans in order to operate our own country. In other words, the increasing loan payments the government continues to make to foreign banks is consuming the federal funds we need to take medical care of ourselves and potentially preventing us from adopting similar government assisted quality veterinary care for our family pets. Federal financial assistance and increased animal cruelty laws are needed to safeguard the care of dogs and cats!

Currently, animal cruelty occurs with pet owners, animal care providers and even city government.

Recently, during morning appointments a mother, daughter and a police officer barged into my waiting room with the daughter's 5 year old intact male Pit Bull, who was in urgent need of veterinary treatment.

According to the officer, she confined her dog to her car too long and the dog was hyperthermic. The dog presented with a rectal temperature of greater than 108 degrees, unconscious, with an overly rapid heart and respiratory rate. The mother left a deposit so that I could start immediate care which included I.V. fluids with added medications and ice packs applied to the dog's body surfaces.

Two hours later, the body temperature, and the pulse and respiratory rates were normal, when I discovered projectile diarrhea containing what appeared to be canned soup with noodles.

Lab work indicated hepatitis and hypoglycemia (32). The dog had to be discharged later the same day because the city took possession of the dog since the owner was indicted on animal cruelty charges. This dog was just starting to regain consciousness prior to discharge and should have had a hospital stay long enough to ensure sufficient recovery.

Instead, the dog was released the same day to be held in a cage at the city pound where there was no climate control or treatment available, because the city, who is now the animal's guardian, is not willing to pay for any veterinary treatment. Now we have animal suffering caused by city government until they arrange to have the dog euthanized or adopted. Waiting for a new owner to accept responsibility for the payment of veterinary treatment is unreasonable, or euthanasia by the city as a treatment to end treatable animal suffering is cruel an immoral. In these types of cases, the chance of anyone adopting a sick dog is impossible so the city orders euthanasia just as soon as they can command the local veterinarian on their payroll to do so.

The federal government also needs to expand the interpretation of animal cruelty laws to improve city and county government conduct. The ultimate priority for the veterinarian that manages the operation of a government shelter is to decrease the euthanasia/adoption ratio. The outcome of this case was in violation of that goal. But lets be fair to this veterinarian.

In order to hold veterinarians employed by city and county government accountable an adequate budget, must be provided to support the appropriate environment, equipment, supplies and staff necessary to take quality care of these orphaned dogs and cats. A deficient budget is the cause of poor care.

Specifically, their responsibilities include management of employees, volunteers, budgets, practicing veterinary medicine and surgery, promoting animal related public safety of the citizens and humane treatment of animals housed, maximizing live outcomes and minimizing euthanasia whenever possible. The salary for such a veterinarian is a meager 70-90k annually.

This kind of low salary does not attract veterinarians with higher levels of expertise whom prefer to work where there are customer willing to pay for their life saving expertise and where they can earn at least twice the salary. Increasing the budget allotted for government services to take care of these dogs and cats will solve the problem.

A larger budget will attract more highly skilled veterinarians and technicians, and create a state of the art working environment with all necessary supplies. This will produce higher quality care.

A higher level of care will ensure that more dogs and cats receive treatment and become adoptable. Additional funding for city and county government for verterinary care will stop many cases of animal suffering and/or cruelty. More funding for the city dog warden should stop another cause of unwarranted euthanasia too.

When there is a dog bite to a person or dog, rabies law dictates what protocol is to be followed. The warden is instructed by statute to provide a quarantined environment or euthanasia for dogs as required. But the warden in an effort to stop unwarranted or city euthanasia, has passed his duties on to owners and veterinarians to save the city money, because owners can not afford the cost of government quarantine. In reality, dog wardens will recommend euthanasia for owners incapable of paying the cost of city quarantine or unable to provide home quarantine, because he doesn't have enough funding to do as the statute dictates on his premises.

Mrs. B called to ask me to put her brother's dog to sleep. Since her brother went to jail the dog bit the pizza delivery boy. She indicated the dog was current on Rabies vaccination, but the dog warden required her to house quarantine the dog or have veterinarian put the dog to sleep. In addition to endorsing premature euthanasia which should be defined as a source of animal cruelty and/or suffering, fundamental mistakes have been made by the city dog warden.

Quarantine is supposed to be done with the dog warden, and if euthanasia become necessary the city employs veterinarians for this purpose on their premises. Any potentially rabid dog is supposed to be handled with the utmost caution by a dog warden and held in strict confinement to prevent any health risk to the public. Promoting home quarantine and an epidemic, and hasty outsourced euthanasia has saved them money, but put the health of the human and pet population at great risk. This situation clearly dictates a legal action by the city to quarantine the dog for public safety, not a medical decision by the private veterinary community for premature euthanasia because the city won't pay for quarantine. A government agency must be designed to check for dog warden compliance with the laws already in place, and a budget designed to include sufficient funds to pay for quarantine and the services of city employed veterinarians. Not receiving payment by the responsible pet owner or funding by the city for city quarantine should not be an excuse for not following the law or insisting on premature euthanasia. Euthanasia because a dog will not receive treatment paid by the city, or because the city will not pay for quarantine is unacceptable. A law needs to be enacted to improve city conduct and stops these types of animal cruelty. This in turn should improve pet owner conduct. Mrs. B should not have to immediately consider euthanasia under these circumstances. Like wardens, pet owners are given too much liberty to exhibit poor conduct.

Animal creulty can begin when an owner simply chooses not to spend money for services.

Very recently Ms. PL came in with her bichon. She claimed that she skin scraped and found mange on her Bichon and her other two dogs that were ailing from similar skin disease. She read on line that it could be mange and she thought to save money she would perform the procedure herself and try to identify the mites on her microscope. She claims to have confirmed the diagnosis and then treated all her dogs successfully with a topical prescription medication that she read about on line would treat the condition. She was able to purchase this prescription medication on line from a foreign country. I asked her if is he would have scraped her children's skin to save money if she thought they needed one done to find a diagnosis. She said "no, because social services would pursue her for abusing her children." We can not allow pet owners to have the authority to inflict any pain on their pets including pain caused by skin scraping their pet's skin. This act should be defined as an act of animal cruelty. Veterinarians should be the only professionals permitted to perform these procedures when the physical finding justify the procedure to prevent this type of animal abuse or cruelty. Insufficient funds to seek or complete the veterinary care for any pet is not an excuse for acts of animal abuse or cruelty. Furthermore, in order to remove the temptation for pet owners to perform procedures on their pets in place of veterinarians, we must stop on line prescription pharmacies native and foreign from selling prescription drugs without our authorization.

Approximately three weeks ago, Mrs. L presented a cat who we eventually learned had swallowed copious amounts of dental floss. Diagnosis was not possible after the initial exam because the cat did not demonstrate abdominal discomfort from abdominal palpation, and therefore the cat was not admitted and radiographs taken in an effort to satisfy the owner's concern to not spend any more than necessary on the visit.

Bloodwork was normal and the diagnosis was not apparent for about another week when the owner returned with floss protruding from the cat's anus. By this time the animal was still stable so surgery was performed immediately.

Seven enterotomy incisions were made to detach and remove any apparent floss from the small and large intestines. The patient survived the surgery and was sent home prematurely with explicit post op care instructions. Contrary to preferred protocol, this cat was sent home 24 hrs post op, because by that time the cost of medical, surgical and hospital care had reached her spending limit. The owner was warned post op about witholding food and that more floss may cause another attack and that further surgery may be required . She picked up some medication 5 days post op and said the cat was getting stronger every day and that she was so pleased. Nothing she described about her cats condition suggested that further hospital or surgical care was needed. Seven days thereafter, I received a card saying that the cat had died and she was broken hearted.

If money was not such an issue this cat could have been hospitalized for extended observation and further surgery performed if needed. This cat suffered and did not have a sufficient chance.

Frequently, I am asked by clients, whether any of my four daughters will follow in my footsteps.

My answer is the same each time. I maintain that I do not encourage them to become a Veterinarian so that they will not have to live a life of continued occupational frustration and disappointment for the many reasons I have detailed in this book.

Because whenever we receive insufficient payment to follow our chosen protocols in the animals best interests, results are compromised causing unnecessary disappointments.

Furthermore, the animals are sent home too soon and owners are making incorrect judgments, concerning the animals prognosis. The veterinarian, not the owner need to determine diagnostic and treatment protocols, and the prognosis to prevent animal cruelty.

If this cat received further hospitalization and surgery, she may have lived many more years. In any case, she would have suffered much less under my care.

This was not a cancer patient who at best would not survive long after another costly surgery. In that case, the cost of a second surgery would be difficult to justify. Lack of government regulations and financial support for our services has kept us from doing our job at the risk of animal cruelty for the hypothetical skin condition with Ms. LP's dogs, and completing our job to the best of our capability for owners like Mrs. L. In many cases even though I operate a one Veterinarian office with two part time assistants in a modest rental where I own all of my equipment and I have streamlined all overhead as much as possible, I still can not provide the best care to many of these patients at a price owners can afford. The outcome of my most recent patient who swallowed a small toy was more fortunate. In this case the bowel disease caused by the foreign body was limited to one location. One enterotomy incision was made, the toy was removed, the cat was given three days hospitalization and released in stable condition as it should be. The sum for all services was approximately 1350.00. A fee that was conceivable to that owner.

But the American dream of practicing Veterinary Medicine is too often a nightmare, and I find it difficult to deal emotionally with compromised treatment results because our treatment protocols in many cases are not adhered to.

My technician told me how a competitor runs a page in the newspaper with the listing of the monthly average of 35 deaths at their hospital. How many of those deaths did not have to happen? What does such an advertisement tell people about the scope of veterinary services? I suppose that is why some pet owners can deduce that it is fair to ask a veterinarian to put their pet to sleep on request before any diagnosis and prognosis is rendered. Why else do I get so many calls to put animals to sleep that I never examined/diagnosed? When I tell them I am pro life and that I would like to get the chance to save their dog or cat, about half of them shorten the call or hang up on me. Why be so rude as to hang up on me?

They feel they should have control over when it's time to end their pet's life because their decision is necessitated mostly by their lack of financial resources. They usually are not willing to pay fees they can not afford to find the truth to determine a prognosis that could justify treatment for their loyal companions. But I will not ignore the pursuit of a diagnosis and prognosis and come to their financial rescue by prematurely euthanizing their pet. What we should be doing is discussing diagnostic tests and then treatment options.

I made a decision to treat the following cat for a low cost despite the owners somewhat indifferent attitude simply because I have the skills to do so. The challenge as expected is to provide favorable results at the lowest price possible, otherwise I have to contend with topic of euthanasia. In many cases four or five hundred dollars is my budget to save dogs and cats.

The budget was four hundred dollars with is case. This lethargic 20 year old spayed female DLH cat presented Christmas Eve with seven day history of polydypsia, polyuria, decreased appetite and mobility. In house glucose testing revealed 261 and 275, and centrifuged urine sediment exam revealed TNTC (too numerous to count) bacterial rods and WBC'S (white blood cells). Immediate assessment was Diabetes and Cystitis. I paid for Blood and urine testing with an outside lab for confirmation. To keep costs down I did not keep this cat overnight to wait for outside lab results because she was not vomiting and because I wanted to save the owner overnight hospitalization cots.

I sent the cat home with Bovine PZI insulin and antibiotics to treat diabetes and cystitis respectively. Again this effective insulin was not available for purchase. Fortunately, I still had one vial left in refrigerated storage in preparation for the next diabetic. I have learned to keep an extra vial ready, because most of the time this product is not available when I need it for reasons noted earlier. The four hundred dollars was used to pay for inside and outside lab work, Chemical restraint injectible, dispensed medication including insulin, syringes and antibiotic tablets. This cat was saved and cared for at a very fair price.

At the time of payment instead of a simple thank you, she told me that the bill was equivalent to her entire weeks paycheck.
At the time of the first follow up to evaluate urine and blood glucose, the owner said with a smirk "I have only 95.00, can we skip the urine analysis?" Against my better judgement I said I would omit outside lab fees, but need to express bladder to examine it grossly. In house blood glucose was normal and the urine was clearer but still turbid. For the cost of 95.00, I dispensed 10 more days of antibiotic, drew blood for glucose and expressed bladder for a gross exam. in an effort to do my job as it should be done. Blood and urine should have been sent to the lab for another CBC, serum chemistries and urine analysis to view any changes to previous elevated findings including blood creatinine, BUN and glucose and urine WBC and bacteria counts. The next week she gave me more of the same demeanor.

At the second follow up she said " I only have 75.00. Just do glucose test. I donʼt want you to express the bladder". I told her I would not accommodate her demand because I had to send the urine to the lab to see if urine infection had been treated sufficiently. She gave me a smirk again and said "I do not want to pay for the urine analysis"

I absorbed the cost of the urine analysis, did the glucose testing and accepted the 75.00. Owners finances and opinions can pose a threat to the practice of quality veterinary practice with this sort of intimidation.

If government financial assistance was in place this scenario could be avoided.

The urine analysis came back normal and the cat is dealing much better after three weeks. This cat would be dead today if I required her to keep her cat with me for three or four days hospitalization to stabilize glucose level. To avoid any potential complications, I prefer to keep them with me for approximately three days to ensure that the glucose levels have stabilized, but this would have caused the bill to be unaffordable to this client. I took a calculated risk on this case because this diabetic cat wasnʼt vomiting and the owner was very willing to nurse this cat back to health. I have kept follow up visits to a minimum to further keep costs down. But, my protocols continued to be challenged by this client.

Yesterday, seven and a half weeks since I first started treating this cat, was the third follow up to check blood glucose. She did not show up for her appointment, even though I gave her a reminder call the day before. No courtesy after all the generous service I gave at a price she could afford.

Often, pet owners will not admit their financial short comings. Instead, age and suffering are two factors an owner will obsess about when they are seeking euthanasia. A more costly surgical procedure such as fracture repair requiring pins or other internal fixation devices is a good example.

Recently a six month female pit bull was presented by Mr. S. Radiographs revealed a three part fracture of the humeral head at the shoulder joint of the foreleg. The owner after learning of this condition quickly pleaded for euthanasia because he claimed she was suffering. In fact, she was suffering more than necessary because he was delaying the expense of treatment to reduce and stabilize the fracture. These types of joint fractures I refer to a Dr. P a very seasoned orthopedic specialist who usually quotes between three and four thousand for his expertise. For your information, complex fractures above the elbow or knee cannot be cast or in some cases single pinned so the cost for fixation with pins and plates can be pricey. In fact this owner preferred that I amputate the leg assuming the cost was less to save money.

Of course, I discouraged that idea and impressed on him to do the right thing by the animal. I am pleased to say that after four pleading dialogues and nine days this owner finally brought the dog to Dr. P for surgery that required three pins to reduce the fractures to align the humeral head to sufficiently endure the joint related functions it performed prior to the accident. Because the dog was young and repair was possible to reduce the fracture and end the suffering it was impossible for this owner to convince me to amputate the leg or euthanize his dog. The next patient owned by Mr. F. requiring similar treatment was not as fortunate, because the owner intentionally avoided the visit I recommended to Dr. P.

One week later he presented his 13y neutered male LabX presented with a simpler fracture of the humeral head. But this patient also required joint treatment. Recent lab work was normal and the dog was a good candidate for surgery.

More complex pinning was again needed because of joint involvement, and to ensure the best quality work I again recommended

Dr. P. At this point I need to mention that many Veterinarians do not get involved in these more complicated types of orthopedic procedures and prefer to refer them to those with much more orthopedic experience to ensure the best care and client satisfaction. For your information, I do welcome fracture repair cases that involve simple pin placement for simple two part fractures where there is sufficient space to securely fixate a pin. But even these cases that can cost as little as $1200-1500 cause too much financial burden for too many pet owners.

Mr. F was shown the radiographs and given Dr. P's name with a strong recommendation. Mr. F told me he would visit him and keep me informed. In fact, he saw how happy the dog was to see him when he was discharged and admitted that the dog was otherwise healthy.

Two days later on a Sunday he left me the courtesy of message indicating that he brought the dog to another veterinarian and the dog was euthanized.

I called Dr. P's office to see if he had brought the dog there for a consult and he did not.

Eventhough the dog was otherwise healthy, the owner wanted to euthanize this dog simply because he was older and he didn't want to pay to fix the problem. Owners will go to lengths to create excuses why the cost to fix the problem is not justified, including once again finding another a veterinarian that renders the treatment decision they choose which is to euthanize their pet. On a Sunday, when I do not pick up the phone, and instead refer to the covering emergency hospital, the owner left me a message implying that he brought the dog to the veterinarian I recommended and without radiographic proof he said the vet told him that "there may be cancer in the back legs, and since the dog was thirteen surgery wasn't a good idea to repair the fracture."

HOGWASH.

I examined the back legs, and showed the owner how healthy and strong they were and clearly pointed out that the dog was an excellent candidate for the surgery.

Very recently, two different owners presented dogs that needed leg radiographs to rule out fractures and I was not given the opportunity to confirm a diagnosis due to lack of a very modest amount of funds for payment. The first was a 15y old Pomeranian that had severe lameness on her left foreleg.

My findings on palpation justified radiographs to rule out fracture of the proximal one third of the radius and ulna. I explained that I would pin the leg affordably if the joint was not involved, only after further communication and consent.

The owner would not pay for the radiographs/development and evaluation at an approximate cost of only 125.00.

Instead, she said she wanted a second opinion, at which time I told her that she hadn't given me the opportunity to formulate a first opinion.

The second was a 10y spayed golden retriever that needed radiographs of his right hind knee to include the distal femur and proximal tibia. She cried and said that she loved the dog but could not afford the same payment for diagnostic films. She too wanted a second opinion at which time I told her that she had not given me the opportunity to arrive at a first opinion.

Both owners left the office with instructions to get radiographs of the affected areas described as soon as possible and neither returned to my office or any where else to my knowledge.

Why does this happen ?

I explained that I am a seasoned practitioner ready to help them at the most reasonable rate in our area, but they can not even afford to diagnose the condition. What is the point of veterinary services, if they can not be rendered. My experience in these sorts of cases, is that both owners will seek the sort of veterinarian that will euthanize both dogs without an accurate diagnosis and prognosis.

I am sorry to admit this, but there are many veterinarians that will do this just to receive some income including additional profits made from selling private cremation services to the owner. Laws must be put in place to put owners and veterinarians on the defensive for this sort of conduct. But without a source of federal or state financial assistance first it will be impossible to enforce these laws in many cases where owners are income deficient.

If there was government subsidized health insurance for these pets, the cost to the consumer could have been reduced sufficiently. Funds would have been available to diagnose and treat simple and joint related fractures, and the dogs described would be alive and well today.

Maybe if gasoline hadn't risen to the price of 4.00 per gallon and heating oil wasn't approaching 4.25 per gallon these owners could have afforded to take care of their pets. The practice of veterinary medicine and surgery is stymied by the lack of government financial support.

The cost of unsubsidized veterinary services should not justify euthanasia.

Veterinary orthopedic specialists such Dr. P are needed . They can only generate their income by performing these more complicated procedures for a small population of more affluent clientele. Most pet owners can not afford the costs of any of these orthopedic surgeries.

These specialized "orthopods" are entitled to the additional fee they charge because they are providing a life saving specialized expertise that took years of dedication and general practice

income sacrifice to develop. To my knowledge, until more
recently, Dr. P has never had the convenience of his own office.
He could not generate enough profit to provide his advanced
skills in one place. In order to find affluent enough clientele for
his services, he has had to travel at great lengths around the state
and get permission to perform his surgeries at the other referral
veterinarian's facilities. It is very possible that he has had to pay
a form of a finders fee to the owner of those facilities when they
are used, which adds to the cost of his services.

More recently at the age of 70+years old he has joined a large
group practice and still depends on referrals from veterinarians
throughout the state. Now he hopes that in his remaining years
as a surgeon, that his long and respected career reputation will
encourage pet owners to drive to him.

He will be sadly missed when he finally retires. He and I have
to over sell his services to clients who frequently overly complain
about the cost and even the driving time to his shared office,
instead of show appreciation for the level of his caring and
expertise. Appreciation for our services starts when we are children.

Some children's poor opinions of our work are unjustly affected
by their parents lack of caring or financial resources to support
our efforts. Lack of financial support for our services causes the
non recovery of pets because they do not receive adequate treatments. Children whom grow up with this sort of exposure formulate poor opinions of our capabilities in the long term for the
wrong reason.

During the Christmas holiday season I met up with a family out
shopping for alcoholic beverages who had a cat under my care
who recently died two days after discharge from my hospital.
This family could not afford to leave the cat for an extended stay
as I strongly recommended so that I could stabilize his condition. Their bill was approximately 800.00 thus far.

Three more days of hospitalization and treatments for a quote of another 300.00 could have made the difference. Oddly, on this occasion the father introduced me enthusiastically to one of his daughters who he indicated wanted to be a Veterinarian. At that moment she glanced at me with fear in her eyes and shook her head no.

Why?

Because she had been disillusioned. She doesn't know that her parents denied further treatment against my advice for whatever reason. She doesn't know that her parents decision to deny further care probably compromised the outcome. Is it my place to point out to the child her parents shortcomings as pet owners?

No.

Apparently the money could be spent better elsewhere including the liquor store. Buying liquor, beer or wine for the holiday is more important to the parents than saving their family pet's life for the holiday.

The child walks away after a sad ending that probably would not have occurred if their was government assistance, laws and programs to protect our family pets just as there is to help the aged or lower class earners. This sad ending sends a message to her that veterinary care is of questionable value because deeply caring for the family pet is not a requirement in our society. Because of this truth, her dream of becoming a Veterinarian and mine to continue practicing is diminishing. We are so enabled as practitioners to remedy many diseases, yet so disabled by a lack of public and financial support. We claim to love and appreciate our pet's loyal companionship, yet deny them the respect they have earned and deserve.

Government needs to intervene to cause people to make the morally correct decisions to properly care and therefore respect these pets. This intervention is needed to promote proper conduct and therefore provide a healthy example for children whom are the future leaders of our country. Ultimately, a lack of perseverance by owners to pursue treatments due to insufficient funds is creating the illusion that we can not successfully treat more complicated diseases.

A few months ago I was presented a middle aged neutered cat with a long history of a blood tinged nasal discharge. Apparently, he has suffered a sinus infection as a kitten that has never resolved. The owner had tolerated this condition as it was until recently when blood began to discharge more voluminously. He went to another Veterinarian in town whom referred the cat elsewhere for a biopsy with no conclusions and now the same Veterinarian was trying to convince the owner to pay for a costly MRI at another venue.

A previous Vet. had taken a subcutaneous biopsy from the forehead of the cat where he suspected there might have been a lesion with a tract to the underlying frontal sinus. The owner was displeased with the results, costs and current confusion, and the care for this cat was now my responsibility.

I anesthetized the cat , determined there was no communication between the biopsied area and the frontal sinus, and closed the superficial biopsy hole left by the previous procedure. Then I flushed the nasal sinuses rostrally and found that the noises on respiration diminished. The cat was sent home with prednisone and antibioitic. and I asked the owner to report to me with advice after two weeks. After a follow up exam I determined that there was no evidence that the antibiotic was an asset to the treatment protocol so I instructed the owner to cease the antibiotic treatment at the end of he third week, but as always I instructed the owner to call me if there was a change for the worse. Thereafter, I did not hear from the owner for approximately four weeks, when he called and said that things had gotten worse. I immediately scheduled the cat for an appointment.

On presentation there was an obvious swelling on the forehead and a tremendous amount of purulent blood tinged nasal discharge. I sent him home with the same antibioitic and prednisone as treatment and asked him to call in a five days so that we could evaluate treatment results.

He called after about two weeks and said he was not able to dose the cat orally as ordered and that the cat's condition had deteriorated and was coaxing me to euthanize the cat. My reply was to admit the cat so that I could administer medication and make any further evaluations as necessary. I told him that since the cat wasn't receiving the medication that it was difficult to justify euthanasia. He was disinterested in my idea and brought the cat to the previous unsuccessful vet. for sympathy, euthanasia and to save money. Again the owner will seek out a veterinarian that gives him the treatment answer he wants. These veterinarians will not make an argument for life saving treatment when there is no type of payment possible for that effort.

If I was given the chance to admit and pursue and evaluate treatment on this cat he may have responded to antifungal therapy. A second deeper biopsy at this time would have been more helpful than the first superficial biopsy done by the previous veterinarian to determine the cause. The main reason why this cat didn't stand a chance is because there wasn't government financed animal insurance, or tax deductions available to the owner. The owner could not afford to leave the cat with me for further hospital care to evaluate a response to antifungal treatment as a second choice. By this time he had spent as much as he was willing to on this cat. Ultimately he walks away thinking that we're not qualified to solve these complicated cases, or that the cat is untreatable because of financial limitations. The fact again is that without government financed support we are not financially able to diagnose and treat many diseased animals that could receive successful therapy.

Without government financed assistance we can only help animals that require only the simplest diagnostic and treatment plans that yield immediate favorable results. Longer periods of time are sometimes necessary to diagnose and treat a condition raising the cost of the services. Currently, in these cases, unless some of the increased costs required to help some of these extended care cases are absorbed by my office as charity, these animals do not have a chance. The public has come to expect some charity with these extended care cases as well as for stray animals they adopt. For stray animals, some people just expect us to take on the additional expense of charity work.

Recently, during evening appointments an older couple I have never met rushed into the waiting room with a stray cat that they had just run over with their car. I allowed the interruption under the circumstances. My first question was if the cats was theirs. The answer was no.

Then I asked if the cat had a Rabies tag or other means of iden-tification so that I could find the hospital and or owner of the animal. Again the answer was no.

Then I explained that I needed owner authorization or a respon-sible party to consent and pay for treatment in cases when the owner can not be identified. I explained further to him that if the owner was to find the cat missing and learned that I treated the cat without their consent there could be a problem for the both of us.

In short these people didn't want to accept responsibility or spend any money for me to help this cat, but expected me to perform whatever treatments I could be liable for at my expense, as well as put off the client scheduled waiting for her appointment. Because I did not choose to treat the cat under the circumstances at my expense, he then turned around and with a disrespectable manner said to this old client waiting for her appointment "You 're going to let this "guy" care for your animal that won't do any-thing for this cat." I suppose he may take every opportunity to slander my reputation whenever possible because I wouldn't attempt to perform services under the circumstances. As much as I sympathized with the driver and the cat's dire situation, I can't ignore the ramifications of treating an animal without consent or financial reimbursement to cover expenses.

I explained to this person that if the cat was wearing a Rabies Tag or other means of Identification that this situation could have been prevented. Furthermore I added that cats should not be roaming free outside where accidents can happen.

Even though this all makes sense I will be called a heartless Vet. by this person.

He couldn't even wait to leave the office before he started slandering my reputation. Here government reimbursed insurance for "orphaned animals" could have prevented this outcome. This cat could be defined as orphaned and eligible for government assistance because he had no tags and an adult guardian present to consent for treatment. If there was such insurance we would admit these cats without hesitation for immediate care and people would instead respect and value our expertise in these situations.

But let's not pretend that the cost of services is the only reason why pet owners do not own up to their responsibility as good guardians for their animals.

Yesterday, I received a phone call from a women I've never communicated with who indicated that she couldn't reach the shelter, which provides very limited veterinary services, after numerous attempts to have her dog put to sleep. She said that the dog has had dental disease since she adopted him from that clinic three years ago, but it has become so bad now that the dog is lethargic and not taking care of himself any longer.

She said she has been aware of the problem the entire time but that because she was on a "fixed income" she couldn't afford to take care of the situation.

The woman claims that she had not secured veterinary care because she was told all the teeth would have to be extracted.

What a ridiculous statement.

As Veterinarians, we do not remove all the teeth as if we intend on placing dentures. We extract whatever teeth need to be removed and remove plaque and tartar from the remaining teeth.

It is obvious to me that she never received professional advice after an appropriate office examination.

I kindly asked her to make an appointment for an exam instead of euthanasia so that I could render a plan if possible to save her pet. She then said he was thirteen years old. I replied that I frequently do dental extractions on dogs at least his age whom go on to live pain free productive lives for years.

I should have reminded her that the dog was ten years old when she first observed and began to neglect the situation. But, let's face it, she didn't make an appointment because she doesn't choose to care for the animal beyond room and board. Apparently, her pet is "just a dog". Shelters can be the "cheap way out for pet owners whom choose to neglect their pets.

A 9 year A/M (altered male) DMH cat presented with a three month history of leaving large volumes of urine outside the litter box. The owner was convinced that these incidents were not accidental, and instead were intentional by his cat. He wanted me to euthanize the cat because he could not tolerate any more intentional urine soiling on his floor. On the contrary.

Clinical findings included an enlarged bladder, difficulty expressing the bladder without anesthesia & catheter and numerous triple phosphorous crystals found in centrifuged urine sediment. The lab confirmed that this cat had urine laden with crystals which typically cause accidental voiding.

The cause of urine found outside the litter box was definitely due to urinary incontinence which is a medical, not a behavioral condition. I kept the bill to 359.00 to diagnose and treat the condition in hopes that the owner would be more interested in keeping his cat.

The diagnostic treatment plan was I.V. fluids and a diuretic injection to fill the bladder to make collecting a urine sample possible, anesthesia to pass a urinary catheter to open a narrowed urethral lumen so I could express the bladder, anti-inflammatory and antibiotic injections, microscopic analysis of urine sediment, payment for urine analysis confirmation at the regional laboratory, and three dispensed medications to commence treatment at home. The owner refused to run blood work on the jugular blood sample that I obtained against my recommendations claiming he was trying to keep the bill as low as possible. The owner was not pleased that I found a very treatable condition with a good prognosis. In fact he still wanted me to euthanize the cat because he did not want to deal with urine accidents during the cats convalescence. He did tell me that if it was his main coon cat he would endure the treatment period.

It is quite obvious at this point that this is "just a cat" to him..

That evening, he left me a voice message and said he would bring the cat to a well known shelter for euthanasia If I wasn't willing to accommodate his repeated request. Some shelters have the lead the public to believe that if a disease occurs that a pet owner can not manage, that they can be summoned to euthanize their pet. If this treatment alternative is an option, then pet owners can choose this cause of animal cruelty. Pet owners should be prosecuted for this conduct.

May I suggest that before a shelter put an animal to sleep that they be required to have a diagnosis and poor prognosis from a veterinarian, instead of make determinations based on the here say of pet owners. Keep in mind that shelters usually do not have the expertise, equipment and budget to diagnose and treat many diseases. For this reason animals with a good prognosis can be euthanized at a shelter to accommodate an owners request. Obviously dogs and cats with unmanaged diseases are not adoptable.

Shelters need government assistance to have sufficient budget to hire the expertise, purchase equipment and pharmaceuticals to care for a wider array of diseases to stop unwarranted euthanasia and stop bad owner conduct. Sadly, low cost private operation conduct can mimic poor shelter conduct for the same reasons.

They pretend they're a full service operation to selfishly generate as much income as they can in the moment. This action can cause the owner to ultimately incur higher costs, while their pet does not receive timely and appropriate services, which increases patient morbidity and even mortality. Recently, Mrs. C called me to schedule overdue dental work on her inappetant cat who was given a long course of antibiotics by the same low cost provider that delayed a referral for dental extractions. The severity of the cat's condition had already caused the animal to refuse nourishment unless antibiotics were dosed.

In addition to allowing delayed animal suffering by not performing or referring the pet for the dental procedure, the low cost center contrary to their low cost promise, compromised the owner financially.

They charged her double the cost that I would have for pre-op blood work and created charges for an unnecessary long round of antibiotics that were dispensed without any intent of performing the dental surgery. The owner had no clue that they never had any intent of performing the procedure. The personnel at the same low cost clinic also told this client that all the teeth would have to be extracted.

It is impossible to determine the need for that course of action without first anesthetizing the patient and removing all the tartar and plaque so that a thorough examination can be done. They obviously were not in the position to render such an opinion.

The public must be informed that typically, low cost facilities are only prepared and able to perform simple juvenile spays, neuters and some vaccinations.

Two days before I scheduled the overdue procedure, the owner stopped by this low cost facility to pick up a copy of her blood work because they could not be reached by phone. They again offered to sell her more antibiotic to generate more income which would have given the owner the potential option to further delay the procedure and further exacerbate her cat's condition. The owner denied the medication, because by this time I had made her aware of the situation.

When the government provides financial resources to pay for veterinary care to assist the poor and middle class and when the government steps up animal cruelty legislation is when pet owners and professionals will improve their conduct. Just as government subsidized health insurance and the Dept. of Child Services was needed to help teach parents how to take proper care of their children, government veterinary insurance and a Dept. of Pet Services (DPS) is needed to be put in place to make sure pet owners take proper care of their animals. When payment is possible for the treatment of choice, there will be no justifiable reason for any veterinarian to choose any other choice of treatment.

Until then owners will try to encourage euthanasia prematurely rather than learn to pursue a diagnosis and prognosis. Imagine if people were routinely euthanized for dental disease or any other treatable diseases like hyperthermia to end their suffering.

Recently, Mrs. K telephoned about their 12 yr. spayed Pit Bull who she wanted euthanized. She claimed she was urinary incontinent, loosing a lot of weight and growing a mass at the right shoulder for the last three weeks and that she decided there was nothing left to do to help her. I said I would look over the record and call her back. I discovered that I hadn't seen the dog for approximately 15 months and found there was no indication to adopt a grave prognosis without an exam and further diagnostics especially since the records did not indicate any compromising diseases thus far. Mrs. K called back three or four days later and scheduled a Saturday exam the next day. She decided to let me have an opinion, unlike Mr. K who was not open minded.

Before, during and after the exam on Saturday, Mr. K insisted the dog was dying of bone cancer and that her condition was terminal. He claimed that one of their previous Pit Bulls had similar signs and that he was certain his dog was dying of the same thing and that was all their was to it . The "Big E" (euthanasia) was clearly on his mind. After palpating the area, I told him that the non painful soft tissue swelling at the right girth which included edema was not attached to the bone. I demonstrated the pitting edema to him and he still wouldn't believe me. The swelling was severe enough to compromise the motion of the right forelimb and cause the dog to have difficulty moving about. Incidentally, the 90 lb.dog had only lost three pounds in the last 15 months. I explained to him that it's more commonplace for a dog who is having difficulty ambulating to have urinary accidents in the house because he can not move about easily, rather than urinary accidents because he is incontinent.

Finally, he admitted he didn't have the money to treat any condition, and I replied that I do not perform euthanasia on command, and that his financial status should not interfere with diagnosing the animal's condition and determining the prognosis. I also told him that I needed to determine sufficient reason to perform euthanasia, because I also have to answer to God's expectations. Furthermore, I explained that after twenty odd years of practice, I stood a better chance of assessing his dog's health status then he did .

I offered, that since money was very tight, that I would limit my diagnostic protocol to radiographs of the shoulder, humerus and ribs in the area of the swelling. Because I charitably kept the bill to a total of 225.00 including medication I had the chance to prove to the owner on the radiographs that their was no bone involvement and that the swelling was in fact soft tissue and edema.

The wife came in two hours later, without her husband to view the radiographs and pick up their dog.

I sent her home with medication for an inflammatory non-infectious injury and told her that I would schedule surgery if necessary to remove any potential underlying soft tissue mass after sufficient inflammation and edema subsided. I telephoned her in a few days and she claimed that the swelling was not reducing. In an effort to save the dog's life by saving the owner the cost of a follow up exam I decided to add a broad spectrum antibiotic to the dog's treatment protocol to determine if there was a bacterial infection involved, eventhough the findings on palpation did not warrant an antibiotic. She promptly picked it up the same day. However, the next day she brought the dog to an out of town veterinary office for euthanasia. I spoke to the office that received her before she was euthanized and advised the caller that radiographs were just taken and that there was no evidence of bone involvement including bone cancer and that the dog was sent home on medication. I also added that the owner could not yet afford any surgery that may be necessary. The fax I received one hour later from that office implied that I treated the dog with a course of antibiotics, NSAID and lasix without success, and that the owner was not able to obtain my radiographs for a second opinion.

Firstly, the dog never received sufficient medical treatment including only one or two doses of antibiotic, to cause any significant
reduction in the swelling, and secondly, she never asked me for
copies of the radiographs for a second opinion. Furthermore, she
neglected to tell the next veterinarian that she saw the radiographs
in my office and the swelling did not involve any bone tissue.

In fact, the fax report to me from this veterinarian indicated that
the owner declined radiographs be taken at their office to rule
out bone cancer. The owner lied to the next veterinarian and
managed to persuade him to put the dog to sleep. Again, the
next veterinarian gave her the treatment answer she always
wanted.

I would like to think that the only reason she lied was because
she couldn't afford further treatment, but I know better. In her
case, the fax indicated that she requested a more costly private
cremation of the ashes.

The money to pay for a private cremation and the return of the
ashes could have been spent on treatment and hospital care. The
fact is that she couldn't be bothered or troubled. Maybe if government assistance was available I could have hospitalized this
dog and the owners would not have had to deal with the dog's
hardships during the treatment period at home. Only hospital
personnel are typically capable of dealing with these hardships.
Again, it's often too much to expect owners to deal with the care
of a patient that requires hospital type care.

I am optimistic that when government assistance become available, that pet owners will learn to take proper care of their dogs
and cats. They will welcome extended hospitalization and more
costly diagnostic and treatment protocols so that we can treat
their animals to the best of our capability. Until then, the " I
can't handle the home care," the "fixed income story" and the "I
don't have enough money" will remain as the common excuses
for not caring sufficiently for their pets.

Financial assistance and the DPS will help eliminate the excuses, and many potential animal cruelty charges. I believe that most pet owners will choose to follow all of our instructions and their pets will receive better veterinary health care after the government has stepped in and provided sources of financial relief. Logically it will be difficult to indict some pet owners on animal cruety charges if government veterinary financial assistance is not put in place.

"Owners without excuses" should be the campaign slogan, to get a bill passed to put aside federal tax revenue for animal health care. One source of tax relief for the middle class to help cover the cost of veterinary care, can be founded by simply adding veterinary expenses to a family's medical and dental deduction .

Currently any medical and dental expenses exceeding 7.5% of the Filer's Adjusted Gross Income is completely deductible. Veterinary expenses for dogs and cats should be grouped with human medical and dental care expenses found on Schedule A. When family pets are given equal attention as other family members or help by the Federal Government is when family pets will get the equivalent level of Medical care they require. For example if the family has an AGI of 100,000K per year any medical, veterinary or dental expenses including insurance costs exceeding 7,500 per year should be subtracted from the AGI before taxes due are calculated.

This will encourage animal middle class owners to spend money to improve the health care of all their family members including their pets because they know that financial relief is in sight if they need to spend more money for better results. This would make the purchase of dog carts more possible for the convalescent care of patients recovering from bone fractures and neuromuscular back and limb diseases.

Yesterday I was presented a 12y A/M Greyhound who had a spiral fracture of the proximal right femur treated three months ago by the leading emergency hospital in our county. Nine screws and a plate were put in place and medication and visits thus far has cost the owner approximately six thousand dollars and the pet is now unable to bear weight on the limb. I needle tapped the fluid filled swelling lateral to the hip joint and found serosanguinous inflammatory fluid. There was no evidence of infection. Needless to say, the owners were exhausted in their efforts and the animal was very uncomfortable. I asked if any external immobilization device was recommended or applied post op. The owner said no. He said that they were instructed to keep the animal immobilized as much as possible during the healing period. The surgery was expensive and their hopes were high and no rear dog cart for external immobilization was required. If a dog cart was immediately put in place for the first three months the dog would not have put so much stress on the fixation device (the screws and plate) and this situation may have been avoided.

Because the owners are already jeopardizing their financial security to do the fracture repair work, unless we insist, they will shun the idea of purchasing a dog cart. But if they could look forward to a tax deduction for combined human and pet family medical and veterinary expenses at the end of the year these dog carts would be routinely purchased and used. Would you expect to leave the hospital after a similar fracture occurred to your femur without a wheelchair?

I asked the owner if he would consider a dog cart at this time, but they could not fathom the idea because they had seen the dog suffer enough. They cried and almost begged me to put their dog to sleep. I had no choice but to accommodate their request, more to end the family's emotional suffering, even though I knew that this euthanasia could have been avoided if the dog cart was given a chance.

It is suffice to say at this time that all the cases discussed in this book would have received better veterinary care if government

financial assistance and direction were provided. To start, I suggest that the models used by the government to determine eligi-
bility and appropriate financial assistance and direction for
people health care be adapted to assist in similar government
programs for veterinary health care. The models for pets must
necessitate that financial assistance, animal cruelty laws, and pet
social services become balanced to provide cost effective veterinary care wherever and whenever it's needed while improving
pet owner conduct.

PART III

THE PLAN FOR CHANGE

Federally funded Veticaid for the poor, Veticare for the aged and or retired, and Schedule A tax deductions for the working middle class are the short term goals. Current government policies need reform to include more conscientious care for our family pets, and the private insurance industry needs more government regulations to better control their greedy motives and unsavory practices.

Private insurance companies continually prioritize profits, instead of our need for sufficient expedient reimbursement for all services we require to do our job the best we can.

We as veterinarians are bullied by the private insurance industry.

We have to typically adjust prices and types of services to appeal to the private insurance carrier so that our services and treatments are more adequately reimbursed. As a result, the insurance companies are dictating to us which procedures we need to perform to support our operations.

The amount of insurance reimbursement is also dictating what the client is charged.

The government in concert with knowledgeable practitioners and influential members of the insurance industry needs to step in and provide financial support and guidance to make Human Medical, Dental and Veterinary health more treatment efficient and accessible to all the financial strata's of our society.

The best decisions for doctor care should start with and be controlled by physicians. When government reimbursement is guided by seasoned veterinarians under their employ, adequate reimbursement will be in place for services rendered in a savvy protocol dictated by the doctor responsible for the patient.

Private veterinary insurance (PVI) companies that give very small inadequate delayed reimbursements to pet owners do not work for the majority of pet owners whom need guaranteed money immediately at the time of services. Many owners can not afford routine lab work, fluid therapy and even one night's hospitalization. Under these circumstances we can not even try to stabilize a patient while we determine a diagnosis and prognosis. Instead as previously discussed, owners may leave the office without treatment in place or prematurely consider euthanasia as their only course of treatment, placing us in a very awkward position. We did not become veterinarians to be the "great euthanizers."

In fact, they will abort treatment advocated at one hospital to find another veterinarian willing to put their pet to sleep because they can not afford veterinary care. This is where we as veterinarians can be at fault, but we can not take on the costs for extended veterinary care without guaranteed payment arrangements.

We should never put a treatable animal to sleep to generate income, help an owner manage his finances, or relieve the city government of their responsibility to pay for the veterinary care of animals in their custody. This action causes the public to believe that euthanasia is acceptable as a treatment of choice by a veterinarian, pet owner or city government when there is insufficient funds for a preferred treatment. More animal cruelty laws will have to be created and enforced and a Dept. Of Pet Services employed to get pet owners and city officials to comply and be held accountable for all pertinent regulations. But unless access to higher government financial assistance becomes available to provide timely and sufficient payment for preferred treatments, it will be unfair to prosecute pet owners for misconduct because choosing veterinary care is dependant on sufficiently available financial resources at the time of services.

Just as owners are not financially prepared for emergency services or extended hospital care without federal or state government assistance for themselves neither are they financially prepared for the same reasons for their pets. Can you imagine the outcry if we had human cruelty laws to punish people that did not have sufficient financial resources at the time of medical services.

Just as Medicaid and Medicare provides federal government relief by providing an upfront payment guarantee to human physicians when their clients are financially disadvantaged so should similar programs for their pets be put in place for veterinarians.

To assist implementation of such programs for animals, I suggest we start by calling these programs Veticaid and Veticare. In addition, we must at least include Veterinary expenses as a legitimate deduction along with medical and dental on line one of Schedule A so that the middle class, which comprises the majority of the public, has a chance to help their pet as their other family members when veterinary care is needed. Even with Veterinary care added to line one of Schedule A as is, the middle class, whom creates the majority of the tax revenue to pay for these programs, will still receive no assistance until more than 7.5% of their AGI has been spent on medical, dental and veterinary care and pertinent insurance coverage. As it stands this 7.5% of AGI should be reduced to 3%, because most of the middle class can not afford to spend that much of their income on family health care. But allowing veterinary deductions will encourage more veterinary healthcare and reduce animal suffering and animal cruelty.

Without government aid and deductible veterinary costs, the veterinary profession remains "all dressed up with no place to go" so to speak. In other words, we have the knowledge and the technology to provide the equivalent level of services that the MD's provide, but lack the financial backing they have to make it possible.

Moreover, without government controlled financial backing, we have very limited hope of diagnosing and treating our patients with worthwhile and effective equipment and services as taught and advocated by our profession. Ideally, as a long term goal, to assist in the delivery of these veterinary services, I suggest we enlarge current state teaching hospitals at state veterinary schools to promote pet owners to receive Veticare and Veticaid. Then we can appropriate federal funds for state veterinary hospital care in an effort to improve veterinary health care in those states.

Teaching Hospitals have most veterinary services possible under one roof, i.e Radiology, Orthopedics, Ophthalmology, Dental Surgery, Internal Medicine, etc..

When all equipment and services are under one roof receiving government assistance it will "level the playing field" and cause all the veterinarians and support staff to work together with in house referrals. This will help implement advanced care to the majority of pets belonging to financially disadvantaged pet owners.

In the states without veterinary schools, the federal government in cooperation with state government and altruistic members of the private sector will need to build and operate equivalent large hospitals to accomplish the same objective. These hospitals will need to keep a budget sufficient to provide veterinary care for invalid dogs and cats that are victims of animal cruelty and/or homeless and held captive in city governed holding facilities. City dog wardens will then be able to transport dogs that need hospitalization or outpatient care to these institutions to receive rehabilitative treatments to eliminate animal suffering and ultimately increase the animal's chances for adoption. No one wants to adopt a sick animal. The management of these hospitals must not be manipulated by support from the more influential affluent members of the pharmaceutical or medical equipment industry that may insist on the sale and use of their products at the potential sacrifice of cost effective higher quality veterinary care.

Large venues receiving government assistance will ultimately attract the majority of pet owners whom usually need financial assistance sooner or later, as well as attract a higher level of expertise because more highly skilled practitioners seeking to practice higher quality medicine and earn higher salaries will receive more payment and therefore better income for their services at these venues.

For these reasons, veterinary medicine and surgery should ultimately be provided by large hospitals as we commonly experience with human health care.

These environments will promote efficient affordable and advanced veterinary care because the operations within will be sufficiently funded and directed by government officials including government salaried veterinarians, whose motivation will be to ensure quality veterinary care at an affordable rate to satisfy the interests of the taxpayer.

But in the short term, just as soon as the current typical small independent local veterinary hospitals can receive Veticare or Veticaid payments, or schedule A tax deductions become possible, veterinary health care should improve dramatically.

In small private practice, it has been increasingly difficult for me to practice after 25 years, or recommend this career to future generations even though my practice was selected for the 2011, 2012, 2013 Best of Bristol Awards by the U.S. Commerce Association (USCA), because the delivery of my services and therefore the outcomes from my treatments are severely compromised in the manner I have described.

I look forward to retiring from active practice at my first opportunity so the mounting frustration in my practicing life will finally stop.

Instead of practicing, I have learned that I can do more to improve veterinary health care and decrease animal suffering and cruelty if I can help to establish any types of government assistance possible, and help stop the illegal distribution of prescription drugs by on-line national and foreign pharmacies. Keep in mind that our goal as veterinarians should always be to solve the medical problem. Their goal is to sell you something. Success in both areas will strengthen the veterinarian patient bond which in turn will improve veterinary health care and the quality of life for our family pets.

In fact, the lack of government guidance and financial assistance, which has caused the increasing choice for low cost inadequate veterinary services and the unauthorized purchase of prescription drugs especially from foreign countries, are the symptoms of the veterinary health care crisis.

It is my sincere hope that this book will raise the public's awareness to the veterinary health care crises, increase animal rights legislation, and cause a movement towards the establishment of government funded and directed veterinary health care programs, so that the profession and animals we care for finally receive the respect and attention deserved.

Made in the USA
Las Vegas, NV
02 November 2021